DYSLEXIA AND YOUR CHILD

HARPER & ROW, PUBLISHERS

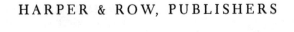

1817   NEW YORK, HAGERSTOWN, SAN FRANCISCO, LONDON, SYDNEY

DYSLEXIA AND YOUR CHILD

A GUIDE FOR PARENTS AND TEACHERS

Revised Edition

Rudolph F. Wagner, Ph.D.

Associate Professor of Psychology

Valdosta State College, Georgia

Published simultaneously in Great Britain by Harper & Row Limited, 28 Tavistock Street, London WC2E 7PN and in Australia and New Zealand by Harper & Row (Australasia) Pty. Limited, P.O. Box 226, Artarmon, New South Wales, 2064.

Library of Congress Cataloging in Publication Data

Wagner, Rudolph F
  Dyslexia and your child.
  Bibliography: p.
  Includes index.
  1. Dyslexia. I. Title. [DNLM: 1. Dyslexia—In infancy and childhood—Popular works. WL340.3 W134d]
LB1050.5.W25   1979   371.91'4   78-4740
ISBN 0-06-014583-8

79 80 81 82 83 10 9 8 7 6 5 4 3 2 1

CONTENTS

• ACKNOWLEDGMENTS

An author can hardly ever complete a manuscript without the stalwart assistance of a host of amanuenses. This book was no exception. Gratitude is expressed to all who have contributed to the successful completion of the manuscript in one form or another.

In order not to disassociate a contributor from his original work, credit lines and acknowledgments have been made in the text where the contribution appears or a reference is made.

During his professional career as a psychologist in public service and private practice, the author has had many opportunities to examine and study hundreds of children with reading problems. Humble thanks must go to these children and adolescents, along with their parents and teachers, for providing the living data on which this book is based. The dilemma of these young people was the motivating force for writing these pages.

R. F. W.

This book was written for teachers and parents concerned with children who, for some reason or another, have a specific reading problem often referred to as a dyslexic condition. The book intends to outline, step by step, how to go about assessing the problem and tutoring a child when no immediate expert help is available to the school or in the home. The approach is not suggested as a panacea; no single volume could contain such an overwhelming task. Nor can the book replace professional help if and when, if ever, it becomes available to the child and his parents.

The message which these pages try to convey to the reader is clear and precise: children with reading disabilities

CAN BE HELPED. While they are most effectively placed in the hands of expert diagnosticians and specially trained remedial teachers, this help is often not immediately available. But until specialized assistance becomes available to the suffering child, someone has to take the reins for ACTION and help the child TODAY and RIGHT NOW! Precious time is often wasted when parents and teachers desperately begin to shop around for professional help, or wait to see if the school system might hire consultants and special teachers—personnel that exist often only in large urban centers or special clinics.

The overt symptoms of a child with a specific reading problem are known to anyone concerned with the education of these children: they are poor readers in spite of good intelligence; they are easily discouraged by their failures; they often reverse letters and whole words; they are sometimes held back a grade in school; they are not disturbed in the pathological sense; they are usually in as good health as most of their classmates; and they have no access to the world of the written word with its literary treasures. They are lost and bewildered in a culture that places a premium on the ability to read. They are often misplaced in society, struggling in the shadow to find their place in the sun. They are called by such labels as Shadow Children, Island Children, Forgotten Children, Interjacent Children, and even stupid children. There is no reason why responsible parents, a devoted teacher, or an enthusiastic tutor could not instigate a well-planned course of action. The book will serve as a first-aid kit and a guide to such action.

The succinct message and mission of this book is one of SELF-HELP by rushing vital aid to the suffering and miserable child who cannot read. Until professional help can be secured, parents and teachers can assist these children by initiating remediation and by providing understanding through emotional support.

Introducing the Second Edition

The problem of helping dyslexic children is as acute today as it was when *Dyslexia and Your Child* was first written in 1971. The need for professional diagnostic services still exists, and an even more crying need for remedial intervention is still obvious. There has been progress in research regarding dyslexic conditions and learning disabilities, but the ultimate "cure" has not been found. Many teachers and parents are still puzzled by the poor reader, with his often colorful symptomatology and pitiful struggle against the odds in school and life.

While the first edition of the book can still be considered very much up-to-date, new chapters have been added to extend its contents and to encompass a wider area of the problem. Thus, the chapter on secondary emotional reactions to learning disabilities treats the subject of the dyslexic child's emotional adjustment more fully. Also, what is going to happen to the adolescent who still shows signs of poor reading and learning? Problems often get complicated in older students because of the chronicity of the difficulties as well as the new obstacles that present themselves. For example, the question of vocational choice in a person who cannot read adequately can take on considerable proportions and calls for critical decisions. Finally, prevention is an important topic that is discussed in the last chapter more fully than before.

New resources have become available since the publication of the first edition, and updated information is contained in the Appendix on reading materials, professional journals, and organizations that offer help to desperate parents and searching teachers. Since the professional literature is beginning to be plentiful, if not unwieldy, in the area of learning disabilities, the terminology and jargon employed in such writings has grown and has confused some readers. For this reason, a Glossary of selected terms used in learning disabilities has been added.

The great plight and desperate dilemma of the dyslexic child is still with us today, but we have made progress over the past decade that has enabled many dyslexic children to improve their skills, get rid of their frustrations, and enter the mainstream of society. To this end, there is hope—lots of hope!

Valdosta, Georgia   R. F. W.
Spring 1979

1 • IS THIS YOUR CHILD?

Children with reading problems can be found in all of our schools and at all age levels. No doubt, the earlier we can detect these problems, the better for the child. Many reading problems in childhood and even in adolescence go unnoticed, only to become a sudden shock to the parents when finally detected and labeled "poor reading" or "specific reading disability." Often the child is held back one grade in order to allow him to catch up with his peers. But while such a measure might be justifiable from the teacher's standpoint and tolerated by the parents "in the child's best interest," the youngster usually suffers agony and feels hurt. He joins children one year younger than he; he is set back. Instead of receiving specialized help with his reading problem, he is exposed to the same kind of instructions he already had in the previous grade; thus he becomes bored, listless, and resentful.

Regardless of the age of the child at the time he experiences problems with reading, many signs of an impending failure are very characteristic and can be detected early if both teachers and parents are familiar with them. Many of us know the seven danger signals of cancer, but few people know the danger signals of a budding reading disaster. Let us take a typical child with a reading problem, a poor reader, as he can be found on the benches of many schools, public and private alike. A parent or educator may well want to take a pencil right now and underline the incidents or characteristic signs and symptoms described below, keeping in mind their own youngster at home or a child they know in school. Let's say the little fellow's name is Henry, but he might just as well be called Michel, Ivan, Leonardo, or Fritz. And some are called Susan, or Tatiana, or Gretchen. *Is this your child?*

The baby had been anticipated by his parents with great joy and eager expectation. The mother had entered the hospital a few days earlier than had been calculated by the doctor, but she was ready for the baby as she was rolled into the labor room. Later she was told that the baby was fine, and it looked as if everything had gone all right. Naturally she expressed some concern about the baby's health, since she had not been able to follow the birth step by step on account of the drowsiness she had experienced during anesthesia, but why worry now when the doctor had said the baby was healthy and looked like a fine boy? The father, beaming with pride as he stepped to his wife's bedside, had to agree that little Henry seemed to be a good specimen of a boy, ready to go home in a few days.

Henry grew up like many other boys in his neighborhood. He enjoyed playing in the sandpile in the backyard, and he liked ice cream. He was somewhat clumsy and had difficulty with hopskipping and balancing on the brick fence. Also he seemed a bit backward and immature for his age and was slow when compared with some of the boys living next door. But he looked cute and was a very happy child. Speech came late. He had trouble with some of the sounds. "Stop that baby talk!" Mother would say to him, and Henry went right on saying "wabbit" for *rabbit,* or "banket" for *blanket.* In fact, it sounded cute the way he said it. Some members of the family adopted his "language" and conversed fluently in it. "Vhere my backfast?" Father would kiddingly say in the morning, and then Mother would reply, "Shamble egg wid toat?" "Yes, pease!" And everybody at the breakfast table would laugh.

Later on in Nursery School, which was highly recommended by a good friend of the family, Henry would say "pasghetti" for *spaghetti,* or "aminals" for *animals.* The nursery teacher kept assuring the parents that this was a developmental stage and he would soon grow out of it. Give him time. Next, puzzles and games presented some difficulty for the boy. For example, coloring was messy, and hopping on one foot was somewhat arhythmical and confused. When crawling was called for in a game, Henry would have a faulty pattern and mix up his legs in improper sequence. But he was still a happy youngster and loved both school and teacher. Bright red stars on his first "report card" testified to the effect that he was doing well. When the alphabet was introduced to the class later in the year,

Henry learned it rapidly. He was a bright boy, according to his teacher. Copying letters was different though; here he was again messy, and often would reverse letters, writing "b" for d, "q" for p, or even "u" for n. When at last he was able to recognize his first name at the end of age five, he would write it

HƎΛRY

In first grade his struggle began. Reading came slowly, and he was labeled a "slow reader" very soon. The teacher again reassured the mother that there were others in the same class who did as poorly as Henry, if not more poorly. There was Ricky, for example, the retarded boy who could not read at all. Just give Henry time, his teacher reiterated. Perhaps there could be a budding underachiever in him, or a late bloomer like his father, who readily admitted his own struggle with reading. Even in college the father, an intelligent man and art instructor in a nearby college, had experienced difficulty with reading his textbooks and seldom read a whole article in the newspaper. A glance at the headlines and news pictures would suffice, and there was always the radio and TV to keep abreast of the daily news.

Henry kept right on trying hard. But the mere sight of the primer made him yawn, and once he even threw a temper tantrum when the teacher was pushing him too hard. He now read very slowly and haltingly. He labored over every single word on the page, constantly looking at the pictures for a clue. The word man was first spelled letter for letter, then put together with the greatest of difficulty. M-a-n, Ma-n, Nam . . . what is this word? Reversals of small words were numerous, like "saw" for was, or "no" for on. He would confuse "the" for a and hardly ever notice the final s at the end of a plural word. He held his pencil clumsily with almost the whole fist of his right hand, and sometimes his left. One day a lady came in his classroom and checked his eyes. Afterward his mother was told by the teacher that he had "mixed dominance," but the explanation the teacher gave was confusing to her. Some of Henry's classmates began to call him a dummy now and teased him during recess in the yard. Why couldn't he read like other kids, especially the girls? Many times he would break down and say to his father, "I guess I'm just stupid!" It hurt Dad more than it did Henry.

Something had to be done about the boy's reading problem, both the teacher and the parents agreed now. His promotion to the second grade was questionable, but it was hoped that with the help of a retired teacher the boy could be tutored to bring him up to grade level. Someone suggested that he had not been exposed sufficiently to phonics, and the tutor promptly set out to emphasize the phonetic approach to remedial reading. After all, one must be able to sound out the letters in order to read whole words. It did make sense. Henry's greatest difficulty and struggle were with little words, strangely enough, like the, these, there, those, and them. He was very proud of himself when he could tackle words like refrigerator or alligator. But at other times he would read "baseball" for bat, just because there was a picture of a boy playing baseball on the page. When the tutor had a conference with the mother, she asked if Henry had ever crawled as a baby. Had he? Why had she asked such a question?

Henry's father also got into the act. Perhaps he should take over the tutorial reins and work with the boy at night. One night, when phonic drill cards did not produce the desired results, only tears in his boy's eyes, Father had an outburst of rage, only to switch remorsefully to a man-to-man talk between father and son. The nightly sessions would usually end up in an emotion-arousing battle, and soon the sessions stopped. It was of no use. Strictness and harsh discipline seemed to make matters worse. Praise and candy bars likewise did not produce any tangible results. Henry could not even recall simple words from one night to the next. His forgetting rate was very high. At least half of the words he had read correctly the night before he could not read at all the next day. They seemed totally unfamiliar to him. One night he would master a series of words flashed to him on cards, and the next night 50 percent were forgotten. Reading was obviously not his forte. Spelling and writing were almost equally pitiful. Henry often wished he could do more arithmetic problems with his father, for there he was on par with the rest of the class. An occasional reversal of numbers got him into trouble, like 42 for 24, but at least he was able to grasp working with numbers. His report cards always looked the same:

Reading	F
Spelling	F
Writing	F
Arithmetic	B
Phys. Ed.	A

And there was always a note from the teacher at the end of the report card regarding his conduct. On each successive card the note sounded more serious. What was left for the family to do? Was the school doing its part? Could it be the teacher?

By the time Henry was promoted to the second grade he was only halfway through his first-grade primer, and even here he was on shaky ground. But he was promoted anyway. Words like *the*, *a*, and *then* still gave him trouble. He would either overlook them completely, as if they were not printed on the page, or read them out loud interchangeably. "A book" was "the book," and vice versa. Henry seemed to love his second-grade teacher at first, but soon love changed to hate when she, too, kept "bugging" him about his reading. Not only could he not stand the teacher, but he hated school and everything it stood for.

Meanwhile sister Susie had come along as number two in the family, and Susie was a joy to watch while reading or doing her schoolwork. She was reading like a breeze on second-grade level, even while she was still in the first grade. Susie was proof beyond a doubt that a child can learn to read if she wants to and is properly motivated. Hopefully, as a friend in the father's office pointed out, Henry might be one of those children who have "high potential" but little desire to learn. High potential!—how they hated that expression. High potential seemed to describe someone who was smart but couldn't make the grade in school. Randy from next door was now in the first grade at age six and was already reading fine. Why not Henry? Just why?

The second grade ended in failure and tears for Henry. He was now barely reading on early second-grade level and not ready for the third grade, according to the principal, who had taken time twice during the year to call the boy into his office, asking him to read aloud while he carefully listened and observed. No, this child could not read like the others in the same grade. On top of it all, he had developed into something of a behavior problem: inattentive during class, bothering others in the yard, making inappropriate noises while others did their work, or telling little lies about having lost his books or having been ill the night before. He was really not a bad boy, just lazy and rough.

Henry had to be held back to repeat the second grade. There he looked somewhat out of place among the new second graders and this seemed to give him the status of the "boss" in class, even though he was more embarrassed than ever when he was called upon to read. He was placed in the lowest reading group, called the "Dolphins," which was a camouflage for slow readers. The new teacher believed in homogeneous grouping, and Henry was strictly placed with all the other slow readers in class because he got the lowest score on the Reading Achievement Test. His scores on the intelligence tests also seemed to be strangely lowered when compared with those of previous years, but then he was often unable to read the directions on the test. In the new class he heard the "Dolphins" struggle and mispronounce words; he heard them reverse sound blends and whole words, like "aks" for *ask*, "plot" for *pilot*, and "was" for *saw*. Father again had started with his nightly tutoring sessions, this time trying to be very strict and stern with the boy. Maybe he needed discipline? One night the whole family was upset at the dinner table because the session with the two men of the house had ended up with a spanking: Henry had not tried hard enough to discriminate between the words *the*, *then*, *there*, *these*, and *those*, and Father had just lost his patience over it and called his son a no-good, lazy dumbbell. That resulted in a temper tantrum on Henry's part, and Father in turn resorted to the switch, which he thought had been stashed away for good. Mother was crying, and sister did not know what to say, so she got out her favorite book and started to read and read.

Good neighborly advice was next. Mother's best friend from college days was married to a preacher, a very friendly man who gave advice freely and generously to anyone in need. She tried to speak to him one day after church to seek out his help. A quick solution was not forthcoming, but what about having the boy's eyes checked? After all, maybe he couldn't see the printed page? Maybe an eye doctor or optometrist could find what was wrong. He remembered a child just like Henry who had had this very same trouble with reading. After he got his glasses, the boy was able to see much better, and his grades improved quickly. And heaven knows, one should be preventive with this sort of thing and go for a checkup anyway. After a visit to the eye doctor, glasses were bought and used for a few days. Henry couldn't have cared less whether he wore glasses or not, even though he did not resist wearing them during class. For a while he tried to cooperate by using them daily, since both teacher and parents insisted on it. But the hoped-for improvement in reading did not happen; on the contrary, the D in reading on the last report card changed to an F. F was not just another letter of the alphabet for Henry by now; F stood for FAILURE.

Soon after the glasses were finally broken in the play yard, Henry's mother read an article in a popular magazine while under the dryer in the beauty parlor. The article stated quite authoritatively that there was such a thing as "Specific Learning Disabilities," also called *dyslexia*, and that it might even be attributable to minimal brain damage of one sort or another. Only experts, however, could diagnose such a condition, the article went on. She also read words like *mixed dominance, laterality, central nervous system dysfunction, EEG,* and *strephosymbolia,* all dark mysteries to her, almost Greek. But there seemed to be renewed hope for Henry. After all, new drugs are discovered every year to cure diseases, why not something new for reading problems? If there only were a pill for Henry that could do the trick. Reluctantly she realized—still under the dryer—that expert advice must be sought at any price. Henry was her oldest, her one and all. The child needed help badly. Hopefully it would not come too late.

The article had mentioned psychiatrists, psychologists, ophthalmologists, optometrists, and other professional people who work as a team with a multidisciplinary approach. A call to the principal of the school brought relief: yes, there was a psychiatrist in town and he was in the same building with a psychologist. One would examine him, the other would give Henry "tests." The two men were also connected with a local clinic, The Guidance and Learning Center, and she could take Henry there for a checkup. Her family doctor also agreed that it couldn't hurt to have him seen at the clinic. Their fees were on a sliding scale, she was told.

Even though there was a long waiting list, Henry was seen three weeks after the initial appointment was made. In addition to several hours of examinations and testing—tests that Henry thought were fun to do—both parents were interviewed by a young lady, probably a social worker. The young lady asked a lot of questions, like: Did Henry ever crawl while a baby? Did he skip this crawling stage? Was or is he clumsy? Were there any injuries during birth? Before birth? After birth? Was the delivery normal? Was there sibling rivalry in the home? And many more questions.

Both parents were partially relieved when they were finally told during an interpretive interview that Henry was apparently suffering from an emotional reaction to his continued academic failure. Indeed he had a reading problem, the staff of the center confirmed. And a severe one at that. Hopefully they might find a trained tutor for him or a special education class if the local school system had one. There his condition could possibly be remedied, or at least improved. Special techniques were used with these children, but trained teachers were hard to come by, the parents were told. Unfortunately, no special class was in existence in the town's public school system, nor was there a private school prepared to take a boy with Henry's special problem. Should the family consider moving to a city where there were such facilities? Should the father sacrifice a good job, the mother her friends and relatives in town?

When the parents came home that day after the last interview with the social worker at the center (they had hoped to talk to the "doctor" one more time), they found a note on the kitchen table. Henry had already gone upstairs to bed.

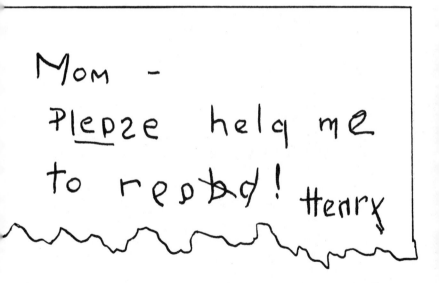

We shall leave this more-often-than-not-true story and case history of a boy with a reading problem. It is the story of Henry—and maybe YOUR CHILD. Those parents and educators who have observed for themselves the plight of such

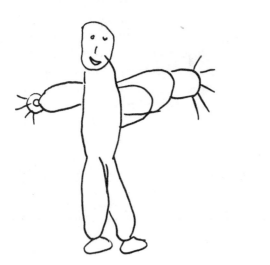
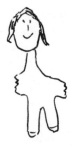

PENCIL DRAWINGS BY DYSLEXIC CHILDREN. Left: *Some of the early signs of dyslexia are reflected in this drawing, done by an 8-year-old boy with average intelligence, mixed dominance (left-handed and right-eyed), and frequent reversals in his writing. In' second grade now, he reads on the early first-grade level.* Right: *Drawing by a 9-year-old girl with average intelligence, immature behavior pattern, mixed dominance, and pronounced obesity. In the fourth grade now, she reads on the early third-grade level. Her reaction to academic failure was overeating and immature behavior (giggling and silliness).*

children are by now convinced that they exist and may have identified with the parents and the teachers of the story. They are indeed painfully aware of their true existence!

2 · WHAT'S THE PROBLEM?

The story of Henry and his reading problem is typical of many youngsters in this country and abroad. Henry had normal intelligence, a healthy body, concerned parents, formal reading instructions in school, a nice teacher—yet he could not learn how to read. If this were an isolated case, perhaps it would go down in educational history as an interesting but rare story of one boy who could not read. But it is not rare, not isolated, not uncommon! It is cold reality that an alarmingly large number of youngsters in this country have this difficulty: a specific reading disability.

Statistical surveys tell us that the percentage of children like Henry ranges anywhere from 3 to 5 percent of the

entire school population in the United States, excluding
the illiterates found among adults, and some surveys place
this figure as high as 40 percent, depending on how the
term *reading problem* is defined and whether or not milder
borderline cases are included. Every classroom teacher can
name one or more children in her classroom who meet the
characteristic descriptions of these children, and every suffering child and his parents make these statistics come
alive. The more severe reading problems will quickly de-
mand attention, even though they go unremedied in many
instances, whereas the milder cases remain unnoticed and
untreated. No doubt the problem has become more noticeable over the past decade because diagnostic facilities have
become more numerous and adequate, but treatment measures sadly lag behind identification of these problems.
Many localities do not have any facilities at all for treatment and remediation.

The child we are speaking of here travels—and fails—
under many names: the Forgotten Child, Island Child,
Interjacent Child, Shadow Child, perceptually handicapped, mild cerebral syndrome, minimally brain-damaged,
slow reader, poor reader, nonreader, stupid, troublemaker
. . . and many other terms equally puzzling to the layman
and confusing to the educator. Professionally used diagnostic categories likewise are myriad and colorful, to say the
least: dyslexia, alexia, learning disability (congenital or developmental), legathenia, language impairment, strephosymbolia, and many more. To top it all, we even find a
fancy Latin name, *amnesia verbalis visualis*, a sort of forgetting visually presented words.

The condition, whatever its name, is very subtle in
milder forms and can easily be overlooked or mistaken for

something else. After all, these are apparently normal children, except for their learning problems.

As early as 1896, W. A. Morgan in England described a case of congenital word blindness in medical literature. Obviously children like this could see with their eyes, but they acted as if they were blind to words on the printed page. They could see a cat running, but they could not read the word *cat*. In 1917, J. Hinshelwood also described the phenomenon in a monograph published in London. Many of these children become early dropouts in our educational institutions, only to begin their painful journey of suffering. Another term used for this condition is *dyslexia*.[1] If the condition refers to a person who cannot write or spell correctly, it is called *dysgraphia*, and trouble with arithmetic calls for the term *dyscalculia*. The first bridges to education were laid by an American neurologist, Dr. Samuel Orton, who thought of the inability to read as a laterality problem, that is, confusion between the two sides of the brain. The short circuits might be caused by the lack of hemispheric dominance in the brain, or in simpler terms, a competition of the two sides, possibly producing mixed-up words and letters, a condition Orton called *strephosymbolia*, a Greek combination meaning "scrambled symbols." All this may sound quite confusing to the reader, whose mind might conjure up scrambled images of all sorts under the human skull. The condition may be hard to describe, but it is real.

The neurological basis for learning problems of the na-

[1] Some dictionary sources give Greek as the origin of the word *dyslexia* from *dys-*, faulty, impaired, and *lexis*, meaning speech, from *legein*, Gr., to speak, but pertaining to words. In this sense, *dyslexia* would refer to reading as well as handwriting and/or spelling, making it a more inclusive definition. Coiner of the term was a German ophthalmologist in Stuttgart, Germany: Dr. Rudolf Berlin.

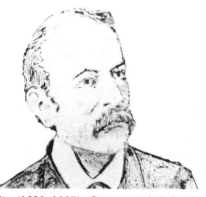

Dr. Rudolf Berlin (1833–1897), German ophthalmologist, coiner of
the term "Dyslexie" (Dyslexia). (Picture from an article by R. F.
Wagner, "Rudolf Berlin: Originator of the Term Dyslexia." Bulletin
of the Orton Society, XXIII, 1973, pp. 57–63. Retouched photo
with art work by Marney Wagner.)

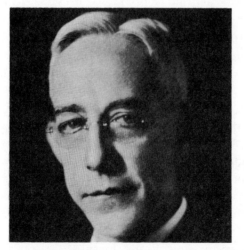

Early pioneer in reading problems, Dr. Samuel Torrey Orton (1879–
1948), American psychiatrist and neurologist. (Picture courtesy of
the late Mrs. June L. Orton, Winston-Salem, N.C.)

ture described here is still under investigation and not fully and conclusively proven. There are many adherents to the neurological model or theory for reading problems, but then they cannot always rush immediate help to the classroom teacher and parent who struggle with the child's dilemma. Regardless of the theoretical speculations or assumed facts, corrective and remedial efforts can only be carried out in the educational setting where the learner's difficulties show up.

If the array of terms has not as yet impressed the reader, there are more. M. Critchley, a British neurologist, uses the term *congenital dyslexia*, implying that children are possibly born with the problem. The developmental aspects of poor reading, that is, the lags and skips of maturational stages during early childhood, are pointed out by still other investigators who refer to this as *developmental dyslexia*. Indeed many of these children frequently show other signs of immaturity in maturational growth and development.

Inferences regarding a hereditary defect accounting for faulty reading have also been made in this connection, because the ratio of boys to girls having this type of learning problem is approximately 4 to 1. The ratio reminds us of the Austrian monk Gregor Mendel, who raised peas in his backyard while carefully observing and recording inherited traits. Mendel's trail-blazing laws often get reinforced when case histories point out that fathers of dyslexic readers admit that they also had this difficulty in school. They would reluctantly admit it to their children, but in the confidential setting of a psychologist's office they often confess readily. Another explanation of this lopsided ratio is the role the male sex plays in our Western culture and the pressures associated with the dominant male role. There are less frequent incidences in the female line of the family, a fact which appears to support the cultural role hypothesis:

namely that women play (or, at least, used to play) a less
dominant role in our cultural milieu. The entire question of
causation or etiology of reading problems is so puzzling that
hunches, theories, and speculations are still the order of the
day, ranging from chemical and genetic bases to assumptions
of underlying behavioral, cultural, or methodological theories. None has completely solved the mystery to the satisfaction of educators and parents, to say nothing about the
child.

The concept of Specific Learning Disabilities is gradually
sweeping across the country and most parts of the Western
world, and has by now infiltrated our educational fields in
guerilla warfare style. The problem has been the center of
much controversy, especially over the last two decades,
among professionals and educators alike. It has also received
impetus through semiprofessional groups and magazine articles in the public and private press. Alas!—the writer found
an article on this subject in "The Bakeshop Weekly" while
traveling in Europe one summer. This paper was handed to
him over the counter, along with freshly baked rolls. And
there are those who deny the existence of the problem alto-
gether but have nothing to offer the suffering child.

The clamor of the throng has by now become loud
enough to be heard by educators, specialists, and the public
in general, all lending a cautious but ever sensitive ear to
the "new" problem that has befallen our children in school.
In professional circles, no one particular discipline is claim-
ing the newcomer: psychiatrists, social workers, psychologists, ophthalmologists, optometrists, neurologists, pedi-
atricians, special education teachers, and others try, in
isolation or in teams, to solve the puzzle. Some take a
serious professional attitude, while others want to make
sure they get on the bandwagon.

In the meantime, parents and interested groups have become quite concerned and alarmed about the problem of reading, for which, apparently, not enough is being done in our schools, public and private alike. Women's clubs and civic organizations have done yeoman's work by trying to inform the public and entice educators into action. They have provided seed money in the hope that once the programs are in the schools and have proved effective, educators will take over the funding. On February 28, 1969, Senator Ralph Yarborough (D., Texas) introduced national legislation, the Children With Learning Disabilities Act of 1969 (S1190). The definition of learning disabilities in this bill reads as follows:

"Children With Learning Disabilities" as meaning those children who have a disorder in one or more of the basic psychological processes involved in the understanding or using written or spoken language. Such disorder may manifest itself in the imperfect ability to listen, think, speak, read, write, spell, or do arithmetic.

Obviously, Senator Yarborough's bill covers a wider range than mere reading disabilities. We note that he speaks of "psychological processes" which may, by interpretation, include learning disabilities that are not primary in nature and were caused by emotional disturbances, for example.

In an attractive folder distributed by the U.S. Department of Health, Education, and Welfare, dated October 1968 and titled "The Child with a Reading Disorder, A Fact Sheet for Parents," the problem is explained thus:

The child with more severe retardation in reading may have problems which are the result of a combination of factors, such as longstanding handicaps of vision or learning, limited general ability, special learning difficulties, emotional maladjustment, or inappropriate or poor schooling.

Significant legislation was passed more recently in Public Law 94–142. Its intent was to bring significant changes in educating the handicapped. This new law is considered the "Bill of Rights for the Handicapped" and covers children who suffer in varying degrees, including the mentally retarded, physically disabled, emotionally disturbed, and learning disabled. P.L. 94–142 was passed by the United States Congress and signed into law by President Gerald R. Ford on November 29, 1975. It is being fully implemented, and its effect has been far-reaching. The new law has four major purposes:

1. It guarantees the availability of special education programs for handicapped children and youth who require it.
2. It assures fairness and appropriateness in decision-making with regard to providing special education to handicapped children and youth.
3. It establishes clear guidelines for management and auditing requirements, as well as procedures regarding special education at all levels of government.
4. It assists the efforts of state and local governments through the use of federal funds.

The law also spells out the rights and protections parents and their children have. It provides for "due process" where the parents' permission becomes an important part in diagnosis and placement in special education classes. It calls for the "least restrictive environment" for the child, including "mainstreaming" where indicated. It provides for individualized educational plans (IEP) that spell out the special education program and lesson plan in writing. The effects of this new law are far-reaching indeed and are still being clarified.

But the more one reads about reading problems, the more

one becomes confused and bewildered. What then are reading disabilities? One thing seems to be true and rather obvious: the experts are not sure as yet. The cold fact remains that some students are unable to learn to read, write, spell, or do arithmetic, in spite of good intelligence, good health, no gross pathology, fair emotional adjustment in the early years of schooling, and a relatively happy home. At this stage of the game some research is going on about these mysterious reading disabilities, but far less than is desirable. The reading disabilities, some experts agree now, are best to be thought of as a syndrome, a cluster of characteristic symptoms. Some believe that at the basis of the syndrome lies a neurological dysfunction, often minimal in nature and hard to detect with the naked eye. What the educator and parents can observe are the behavioral manifestations of whatever causes the problem. While some theorists infer the existence of a brain problem, others refer to it as perceptual dysfunctions not necessarily organic in nature. Then there are those who wish to blame the educational methods used to teach these children to read in the first place. Still others try to de-emphasize the learner and have had a closer look at the writing system proper: if a child has difficulty with left-right orientation and confuses b with d, naturally he has difficulty with reading, but one should not find fault with the learner. It's our antiquated, outdated, outlandish system of writing, which has changed little over the years.

Until all evidence is in, perhaps it is best and wisest to look at reading disabilities strictly from a behavioral point of view, that is, deal with them at the level where they can be noticed and possibly remedied. Knowing the "danger signals" and characteristics accompanying the problem is perhaps the best we have to offer at this point. The best progress, in terms of helping the child, has thus far been made wherever and whenever something was being done about the problem. Being told what type of problem a child has is one thing, but parents want to know what to do about it. Educators are annoyed when someone reaffirms what they already knew, namely that the student cannot read; but they appreciate a person who comes into their classroom and shows them how to deal with such reading problems. Call it by whatever name, THIS CHILD needs help with reading.

By far the most popular household word for the problem today is *dyslexia*, probably because it offers an appealing semantic label for a child's bewildering problem—a term that brings instant consolation to the concerned parents, relief to the struggling youngster, and a halo atop the specialist's head. The term *dyslexia* means a disturbed function of the symbolic and perceptual abilities, manifested in poor reading, much below the expected grade level for a particular age of the child. Once diagnosed, it is up to the educator and methodologist to remedy the dysfunction of the reading process. This is an important aspect of the dilemma, because too many parents and teachers stop with the diagnosis and are at a loss because of a lack of information on remediation. For an analogy, we might think of a disease for which medical specifics have been found to control the disease but whose cause is yet to be discovered in the laboratory. One cannot go on hoping for new discoveries; these children have to be helped HERE AND NOW. Interesting facts pop up from time to time, but they do not find their way into the classroom as rapidly as desirable or in time to help many children. For instance, a research study shed new light on an old problem by pointing out that the incidence of dyslexia is less than 1 percent among children in Japan. Why should this be so? A possible explanation would be that perhaps we have been looking for the causes of poor reading in the human system when actually the symbol system—the writing employed for reading purposes—might be unsuited for the task of reading. Japanese characters do not require a phonetic word attack, and the task of left-right movements likewise is not needed. It is more comparable to our word recognition method or sight reading.

But enough of historical and theoretical background in the midst of a labyrinthine puzzle of terms and nomenclature. What about your child, your student? Why not call him right now, this very instant, and ask him or her to read these simple words to you:

dip was bib split on from bid dud tilt tub stilt

tar for tab dab blend skip crow pelt felt *b* *d* *b* *b*

Could he read all these words and letters without hesitation? Did he reverse any letters or words? These are indeed simple words which a child was exposed to during the early years of formal reading instructions. They were deliberately chosen as veritable "traps" for a child with a severe reading problem. The same mistakes, if any, are also made by young beginning readers in the first grade, and only if this type of faulty reading persists or is excessive must one suspect a severe reading problem. Strangely, some children do not reverse these words and letters but still have a reading problem. They too need help, but their deficient reading stems from a different type of reading difficulty, and will be discussed later under difficulties with auditory discrimination. The older the child, the more indicative these reversal errors are of the existence of a specific reading disability.

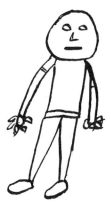

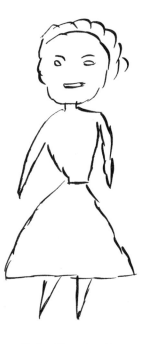

PENCIL DRAWINGS BY DYSLEXIC CHILDREN. Left: *Drawing by an 11-year-old boy, with high average intelligence, difficulty with left-right discrimination and orientation, and poor reading ability. Placed in the fourth grade because he was held back one year, he now reads on the third-grade level. He is shy and withdrawn and has few friends. He is easily distracted and easily forgets words he has studied the day before. Spelling and writing are also very poor. He has little confidence in himself and is disenchanted with school. His medical records show many childhood diseases with fever running as high as 105°F. at one time.*   Right: *Drawing by a girl, age 16, with an above-average intelligence level (IQ 119). Now in the eleventh grade, she is reading on the early seventh-grade level, showing poor word attack and reversal of words. Her emotional reaction to academic failures has made her shy and withdrawn. Her father also had difficulties with reading in school, all the way up to college.*

3 · DANGER SIGNALS OF POOR READING

Many parents may think their child is reading above grade level, when in fact it is only average, or vice versa. Other parents might judge their child's reading skills as rather poor and slow, when in actuality he may read on an average level, when compared with other children in a normal grade. Unless a person is well trained in the field of teaching reading, his judgment will often be colored with well-meant bias and tinged with emotions. This chapter will enlarge on the characteristics of poor readers in order to sensitize the observer's judgment to the typical symptoms that plague the poor reader and the dyslexic child. In the next chapter we will provide objective devices to assess a child's reading skill more quantitatively in terms of actual measurements. And perhaps some readers may not have in mind a particular child of their own, or a special student in their class, but simply wish to seek more information about reading disabilities in order to prevent reading problems in the future and recognize them when they occur. This perhaps is the wisest approach to the problem—preventing reading problems from happening. While such idealistic thinking lies yet in the future, we must realize that the future has already begun! There are many evaluative techniques and teaching methods that are known to the specialist in the field, but are little known to the grass-roots teacher and home-bound parent.

Pioneer work in the field of preventing reading problems has come from Katrina de Hirsch, among other investigators, who studied many young children, both healthy and prematurely born.[1] After giving these children a battery of tests to see just what they could and could not do, and following up the same children after several years, de Hirsch essentially found that poor reading *can be predicted* at an early age, even though not in all instances. Early symptoms of reading problems often go unrecognized when they could have been detected and remedied.

What are some of the danger signals of poor reading that we want to look for? First of all, there are primary characteristics which are directly related to reading, and secondary ones which occur in reaction to the primary disability. They may not be directly connected with the reading problem per se. All together they form a cluster of typical signs known as a syndrome. Of course, nobody can speak of poor reading until the child has reached the age or stage where he would ordinarily be expected to read, or

[1] Katrina de Hirsch et al., *Predicting Reading Failure, A Preliminary Study* (New York: Harper & Row, 1966).

until he has been exposed to formal reading instructions. The label "poor reader" is not attached to the child until he has had a chance, has tried, and has failed. But the early signs nevertheless were there *before* the child ever started to read. Successful prediction is not possible in all in-instances, but concerned teachers and educators will want to look out for these signs.

Characteristic Signs of Reading Disabilities

Primary Characteristics

The reading problem, partially or totally, usually shows up with the beginning of formal reading instructions.

The child shows poor ability to associate sounds with corresponding letter symbols. He knows and speaks the "hissing sound," *s*, but cannot relate it to the letter symbol S.

Details of words are often ignored, i.e., the child has a poor memory for parts of the word and also has difficulty retaining the word in his mind.

Word guessing is frequent due to insufficient skill in word attack. The child may not look at the words but instead seek pictorial and extraneous clues. This habit results in poor reading.

Confused spatial orientation is evident. For instance, a child may reverse letters, words, and numbers. He may have difficulty discriminating between the letters *d* and *b*, or even *d* and *p*. Mirror reading and writing is frequently encountered.

There is much confusion of left and right. Mixed and confused eye-hand-foot coordination ("crossed dominance") may exist but in and by itself does not constitute a basis for diagnosis.

Auditory discrimination is often poor; the child cannot distinguish between words like *pen/pin*, or *dip/lip*, when they are pronounced for him. Hearing, or auditory acuity, is usually unimpaired.

The child may lose his place on the page or skip a line or two.

In addition to awkward coordination, there might be other areas where difficulties exist, e.g., working with jigsaw puzzles, holding a pencil properly, or walking on a chalk line.

Newly learned words are forgotten from day to day: The child may be reading better on some days than on others. Reading rhythm is usually poor and labored.

Secondary Characteristics

There is no mental retardation or below average intelligence.

Discovery of the reading disability comes only after the child has entered school. Before the school entrance, he appears "normal" when compared with other children of the same age.

Dyslexic conditions occur more frequently in boys than in girls, with an approximate ratio of 4 to 1. The difficulty is supposed to be sex-linked genetically because many fathers of poor readers also had reading difficulties in childhood.

General confusion in orientation can be noticed even before the child enters school. He may confuse days of the months, time, distance, size, or left-right directions.

Motor coordination is frequently poor, such as a veering or swaying gait, awkwardness when playing on the playground equipment, or holding the pencil unconventionally.

Speech delays and speech difficulties may also occur, but the child's speech may also be perfectly normal.

Health is usually unimpaired in general. Upon neurological examination, milder forms of neurological dysfunction are sometimes discovered, but no gross pathology exists.

The child feels more and more inadequate as he encounters reading failure. He feels "dumb and stupid" and develops emotional reactions in response to his failures.

Special tutoring with conventional teaching methods has not helped the child in the past; improvement of reading even over weeks and months is minimal and not commensurate with normal progress.

Secondary emotional reactions in response to protracted reading failures show up sooner or later as the child struggles to keep up with his peers. These reactions may take the form of general irritability, aggressiveness, avoidance reactions, defensiveness, withdrawal, behavior problems, and many others.

It should be stressed here that a reading disability usually shows up in clusters of symptoms—one symptom in isolation is not necessarily cause for alarm. However, if any one of the signs described above is very severe, or if several of them exist, professional advice must be sought to pinpoint the problem.

Just what causes these reading problems in children is still a controversial subject even among professional workers in this field. Educators are still more puzzled than informed about the problem, and only in some localities are experts available who may instigate remedial procedures in the schools or reading centers. Some authorities say that a malfunction of the neurological system is at the basis of these problems, while others take issue with this concept and suggest that other factors are operant in the disability. It is not our intent to enumerate and discuss the merit or adequacy of the various theories, assumptions, and speculations that have come up from time to time in the professional literature and popular magazines. It is of little use for the layman to know whether the free flow of a chemical substance in the blood is responsible for the reading failure of a child, or if the antiquated system of our English language is to blame. What is of paramount importance is that we must bring immediate help to the struggling youngsters who cannot read like their pals in class. YOUR CHILD NEEDS HELP NOW!

Two topics will be singled out especially here because so much is talked about them in relation to poor reading: vision or eyesight, and neurological deficiencies. Good eyes and a good nervous system are certainly prerequisites for good reading, but since the process of reading is a multivariate one involving many functions of the human body and mind, their role can easily be overemphasized while other aspects are completely overlooked or taken for granted.

Here is what Dr. Harold Friedenberg, an optometrist and chairman of the Committee on Visual Problems of Children and Youth, American Optometric Association, has to say about vision and reading:

People who equate vision with visual acuity are quite correct when they assume that vision—as they define it—has no relationship to reading. It has been proven time and again that 20/20 vision at distance bears little relationship to reading problems. Refractive errors, binocular problems, fusion difficulties and reduced amplitude of accommodation do not prevent a child from learning to read. Once a child has learned to read, however, these ocular problems may make reading slow and uncomfortable and cause the child to seek out other activities less distasteful than reading. The child with the most obvious ocular defect—a youngster whose eye turns so far in or out that he cannot use it—is rarely impaired in reading because of his ocular problem. Yet the child whose eyes look straight, but do not function together adequately may develop fatigue and discomfort while reading and may not read as rapidly or with as much comprehension as he is capable of because of this ocular or end organ problem. While certain types of refractive errors, particularly hyperopia in moderate or greater degrees, anisometropia—difference in refractive power of the two eyes—and certain types of astigmatism as well as accommodative, fusional and binocular difficulties contribute to inefficient reading and interfere with reading performance, they do not in themselves prevent a child from learning to read. These visual conditions do not give rise to dyslexia, strephosymbolia, congenital word blindness, or any of the other labels currently being affixed to the child who is a nonreader.[2]

[2] Verbatim quotation from a prepared statement written by Dr. Harold

We must realize that reading involves our eyes, but it goes far beyond the eyeball proper. The child has to be able to interpret what he sees, and this is called visual perception, again only one aspect of the total reading process.

In connection with visual perception, the mystery words *mixed dominance* are often heard. Among the theories and methods which take this confused eye-hand-foot coordination into consideration are Dr. Samuel Orton's contributions and the Doman-Delacato method. The subject is controversial to this day, to say the least, and conclusive evidence is still to be presented to the serious researcher under laboratory conditions. This author's experience has taught him that mixed dominance in and by itself rarely interferes with reading, unless other signs and symptoms of a poor reading syndrome also exist. Partial proof for this statement can be found in the fact that many good readers, with average intelligence, have mixed dominance also. If it does exist along with other signs and symptoms of poor reading, however, it seems to further depress the child's ability to read. In other words, it seems to contribute further to poor reading which would exist anyway.

A child's lateral dominance, or sidedness, can be tested crudely by teachers or parents. Hand dominance is established by observing the child as he writes on paper, while foot dominance can be observed by asking the child to kick a ball or object. Testing of eye dominance can be accomplished by asking the child to hold a simple funnel in front of both eyes, with the examiner looking at the aperture facing him to note the dominant eye. Among children, dextrality or complete right-sidedness is the most commonly found laterality, with right-hand, left-eye, right-

Friedenberg, Richmond, Virginia. Dr. Friedenberg's kind permission to quote extracts from his statement is hereby gratefully acknowledged.

SIMPLE FUNNEL DEVICE FOR TESTING EYE DOMINANCE. (1) *Roll up ordinary sheet of paper as shown, leaving hole approximately one-half inch in diameter. (2) Hold horizontally in front of both eyes, with both eyes kept open. (3) Dominant eye will show through hole pointing toward the observer.*

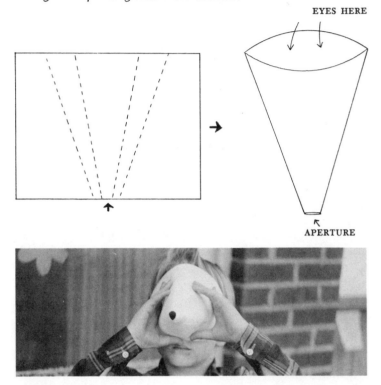

EYES HERE

APERTURE

Hand dominance can be observed by asking the child to hold a pencil and write down a word. Some children prefer one hand for writing, the other for gross motor activities, such as throwing a ball or cutting with scissors. Foot dominance can be observed by asking the child to kick a ball. The child has "mixed dominance" if eye and hand are not on the same side, e.g., right eye and left hand. Confused dominance does not appear to mean anything in and by itself but often contributes to the adverse signs in a reading problem by adding to the child's poor reading ability. Some normal readers also have this confusion in sidedness but seem to be able to compensate for it (sometimes by superior intelligence).

foot being next in order of occurrence. Some children are ambidextrous, meaning that they might prefer their right hand for writing activities and the left hand for gross motor activities such as throwing or batting a baseball. Other combinations are of course possible, but they are rare. The reader interested in testing eye dominance may wish to refer to the illustration for further explanations of the funnel test. The developmental aspect of lateral dominance has to be mentioned here, since very young children may not establish a preference for eye dominance until they reach the age of five or six. Hand and foot preference seem to be established earlier.

Neurological Handicaps Related to Poor Reading

Many people think of "brain damage" in terms of a person with a big hole in his head or major malfunctions of the brain mechanism reflected in grossly abnormal behavior of one kind or another, including nonreading. The subject is of interest here inasmuch as poor reading is linked to malfunctions of the central nervous system. Evidence exists that neurological handicaps in children indeed show a close correlation with poor reading, but not necessarily so. Besides, if this correlation does exist, are the remediation methods different for both conditions, neurological and nonneurological? Recent trends favor treating both types of poor readers with similar methods, possibly modified for individual cases or specifically isolated trouble areas. To make teachers and parents aware of existing organic conditions that must not be overlooked, the subject of neurological implications in dyslexic conditions will be further discussed with regard to their signs and symptoms.

Brain damage can occur not only in minor forms and in various parts of the brain, but it may also show up in a very mild form of borderline degree. Minimal brain damage is also referred to as subclinical or borderline damage (CNS, or central nervous system dysfunction) and may affect one or several areas of the brain, centrally or peripherally. It is rather cumbersome to diagnose and can be done only by the medical specialist after intensive testing and examination. It is usually the neurologist who makes the diagnosis, but the "soft signs" of the condition can often be observed and recognized by alert teachers and parents who can then make the necessary referral to the medical specialist. These signs are also often recognized during psychological examinations as perceptual or coordination problems.

What are some of the characteristic symptoms that teachers and parents can observe in children with this type of difficulty? Again, the basis of observation is the child's behavior, the way he acts at home or in school. There are many signs that should be looked out for, but one symptom alone may not necessarily be significant unless a gross disturbance exists. We therefore speak of a syndrome, a cluster of signs and symptoms, all characteristic of children with neurological handicaps. The very same sign could also show up in other children not necessarily having a brain problem. What are some of these signs?

Poor schoolwork	Overactivity at home and in school
Nervous mannerisms	Emotional problems
Distractibility	Impulsive behavior
Short attention span	Poor reading and spelling
Clumsiness	Destructiveness
Speech peculiarities	Lack of concentration
Confused orientation	Confused writing or spelling
(Space and/or time)	Catastrophic reactions

These are just some of the typical signs. There are others, perhaps more subtle, and they do remind us of the characteristics of poor readers described earlier. The reason for such symptom overlap may be explicable in terms of the variability of the two conditions; neither one of them is considered an entity. There are great differences among poor readers, and there are great differences in children with neurological handicaps.

The developmental history of children with brain problems will often reveal typical incidents of a critical nature. But again, a word of caution is in order. While these incidents are noted, they are by no means significant in every instance. It can hardly be proven after the fact that a mother's pain during pregnancy is directly related to a child's poor reading performance now. Here are some of these typical signs during the child's developmental history:

No crawling during early childhood

Late walking and/or talking

Poor left-right discrimination

Awkward gait or clumsiness

Poor orientation in space or time

Rotation of simple drawings (poor copy work)

Irritability and nervousness

Mixed eye-hand-foot dominance, poor coordination

Frequently mothers of children with neurological handicaps report some incidents related to birth—oxygen deprivation of the infant, use of instruments during birth, prolonged labor, and other more complicating factors before, during, and after birth of the child. Physical examinations of a general nature might not reveal anything unusual; general health is often judged as good. When drugs are prescribed, they may help to reduce irritability and other interfering symptoms. At best they make the child more amenable to learning; they do not cure the learning disability itself.

The schoolwork of these children reveals weaknesses in either the verbal or numerical area of conceptualization and abstraction, manifested in poor reading and arithmetic skills and accompanied by poor spelling and writing. Any one of these areas may show up alone or in combinations.

Initial parental expectancy may be high for the child because parents are unaware of the existence of a neurological problem. They often have normal and above average intelligence themselves, which may at times present a psychological difficulty in accepting a child with a learning problem. The problem is often not noticed or admitted until the child enters formal school, where he has to meet certain academic and social standards in comparison and competition with his classmates. Results on general intelligence tests usually show a high amount of so-called scatter or variability among the various subtests, that is, the areas tapped by the test. The areas which test the child's perceptual ability are usually low, even though the intellectual potential is judged average or above. This may be all the more confusing to parents and teachers. The child is good in some areas, and quite below average in others. There may be islands of brightness in an ocean of academic defeat.

The classroom teacher will initially struggle with the child, trying to offer him an intensified dose of conventional or remedial teaching methods. But the child does not readily respond to these techniques, because we are dealing here with a *specific* disability which is not similar to the ordinary learning problems of the underachiever who lacks motivation and drive, or of the emotionally disturbed child who in severe cases also may present a learning problem whose cause is of a different nature. Poor reading may be regarded as a symptom, not a cause, and it is for this reason that dyslexic as well as neurologically handicapped children may often be found in classrooms for the mentally retarded. The answer to these children's problems is not one of retention or isolation; it must be specific diagnosis followed by specific treatment.

Many authorities now claim that there are several causes for a specific reading problem, and each one may need a tailor-made remedial program. However, in each instance the fact remains that the child is not able to read. It is truly amazing how a poor performance in reading can lead to all sorts of related problems in our culture. And if the handicap is not remedied, severe punishment awaits the nonreader—nothing short of ostracism from the mainstream of our cultural life, including educational advancement, job opportunities, and even recreation.

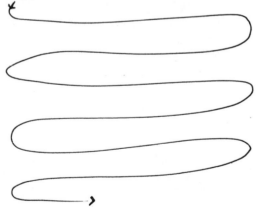

Why do we write (and read) from left to right? *The early Greeks introduced a form of writing that alternated back and forth on successive lines. This pattern was called boustrophedon (literally, "as the ox turns"). The method was the forerunner of the left-to-right reading system used in the Western world to this day.*

4 · ASSESSMENT OF THE PROBLEM

While you know that your child or student needs help with reading and needs it right away, we have first to ascertain just how deficient his reading skills are in order to initiate the proper remediation. Just what is the child's reading level at the present time? Measuring the reading level alone is of course not the sole determinant of a reading problem. He has to have several of the typical signs of a specific reading disability that go with the entire condition. Poor readers exist in almost every school; and if they also are slow in mental functioning or have an emotional disturbance of some kind, below average reading is to be expected.

The first thing we have to know is how intelligent the

child is. It's the baseline. Without going much into the disputed pros and cons of the intelligence concept and IQ measurements, let's use some common sense right from the start. The closest relationship to intelligence is a person's word power, his vocabulary, the words he knows or uses. If a child has a good vocabulary like most of his peers, he should be about average in intelligence. That's why most intelligence tests have a section that tests vocabulary and language usage. Use of vocabulary and the intelligence level are the best single predictors of future academic success we have at the present time. Another way to determine the intelligence level is to call on the child's teacher or school counselor and inquire about Henry's results on the group test he has taken in school. In most states group tests are mandatory, and the results should be on file at the school or central administration. While school personnel will be reluctant to quote an IQ score or percentile rank on a given test, they will usually not hesitate to quote the child's relative standing on the test—average, below average, or above average. And that's good enough for our purposes at the present time. Any precise assessment of intelligence should be done only by a qualified psychologist who is able to administer individual tests and interpret them. We'll get to that later.

Suppose you determine that your child is of at least average intelligence, possibly above but not below average. Mental retardation, usually determined by an IQ cutoff score of 75 and below, among other physical, psychological, and emotional determinants, will not enter our discussion here. A child with low mental ability is also expected to be slow or poor in reading. For instance, a boy of nine, with average mental ability, would ordinarily be in the fourth grade, given good health and adequate motivation to learn.

But if the IQ were below 75, which is considered mentally retarded by most standards, he would probably not have earned his way to the same fourth grade. He is expected to be a poorer reader than his average peers. At the same time, a boy of nine with an IQ of 120—that is above average or superior—is ordinarily expected to be a superior reader even if he is placed in the fourth grade with his own age group. However, as we shall see later, a child with superior intelligence, but reading only at the grade level to which he is assigned by the school, still could be regarded as a problem reader, because with superior intellectual ability he should be reading above grade level. These crude calculations of the expected reading level should give us at least some approximation as to where a child should ordinarily be with his reading. Without the establishment of reading expectancy levels, we cannot determine a reading deficit. Just how poor is poor reading? If the child reads *one or more* grades below his expected reading level, *he needs help!* Owing to developmental stages, the difference between expected and actual reading levels is smaller in the early grades and becomes much more of a gap in higher grades. For example, a boy who reads at the 1.5 reading level (at the end of the fifth month in the first grade) while in the second grade may be as far behind in reading as a boy in the fifth grade who reads on the fourth-grade level. In high school, this difference may be even wider; a boy in the eleventh grade might still be reading at the fifth-grade level, even though he has average intelligence, because of a dyslexic condition.

Here are simple steps to be taken by responsible teachers and parents when they suspect a reading problem. This quick checkup can be initiated by the parents, preferably in cooperation with the school.

What to Do

1. Ascertain an estimation of the child's level of intelligence.

2. Determine the child's present level of reading skills.

3. Find out if the child has some or all of the typical signs and characteristics of a specific learning disability.

4. Examine carefully the quality of the child's oral reading and determine if he reverses letters or whole words.

5. Try to find out where professional help is available if needed.

How to Do It

Based on the five steps outlined above, here now is what needs to be done right away.

1. Contact the appropriate school administrator (teacher, principal or guidance counselor) and ask if the child has been given any group or individual intelligence tests in the past which would indicate his intelligence level. Don't try to pin them down to an exact IQ score; just simply ask if your child is average, below average, or above average, according to the test results. Ask the teacher also for her own observations in the classroom, since group tests are usually verbally oriented, and your child may not have been able to read the questions on the test. The teacher may have some indications that the child actually is brighter than a mere test score can show.

2. Use the simple reading test described in this chapter to determine the child's present reading grade level. The test gives an estimate of the grade equivalent and provides a basis for the so-called instructional level, i.e., the level at which remediation should begin.

3. Go through the checklist of characteristics of children with learning disabilities, also contained in this chapter. Care should be taken that the child is not rated too harshly; objectivity is in order here. Teacher and parent may want to do this rating on the checklist together to obtain the desirable objectivity. There should be several items checked on the list. The younger the child, the higher the number of items might be checked off, since some of the signs

are also characteristic of a normal phase during a developmental stage.

4. Use the Inventory for Reversals in this chapter, described further below, to examine the type of reading errors the child makes. In particular, what needs to be looked at is the number of reversal errors, such as "was" for saw, which are typical of poor readers.

5. Professional resources for diagnosis, remediation, and therapy are described in chapter 5.

A. Administration and Scoring of "Estimation of Reading Grade Level"[1]

Administration of the test (see page 57) is simple and can easily be done by teachers and parents. It ordinarily takes no longer than a few minutes. However, users should keep in mind that the results of the Reading Estimate can serve only as a guide for further exploration of the child's reading problem. The results will serve as an indication of where the child's instructional level lies, and thus where remediation should begin. For example, a boy age 12 and placed in the sixth grade but reading on the third-grade level, should not be tutored on the fifth- or sixth-grade level. Remediation must begin at the level where his present reading ability was arrested, in this case at the third-grade level. The Estimation would also lend itself well to surveying an entire class in order to get an idea where the group stands with regard to reading. The main emphasis of reading instructions for the entire class should then be placed on the average reader in the class. Most schools now use individualized instruction methods, and here too the teacher can use the test results for the necessary groupings.

---

[1] Teachers and other school personnel wishing to obtain information on the standardization of the Reading Estimate, including reliability and validity, should communicate with the author.

After briefly establishing good rapport with the child, the examiner proceeds with the administration by asking him: "Read just a few letters and words for me, please!" and "Read aloud so that I can hear you!" Testing is always begun at the K (Kindergarten) level, on through Grades 1 to 6, and is discontinued after the student has failed to read at least six words correctly, or after he has missed an entire line. The student should be given sufficient time to allow for his word attack, but it is proper to say, "Go on to the next word!" if there is no indication that he will come up with the correct pronunciation within 30 seconds. No prodding is permissible, of course.

The recording of the responses is done on the sheet itself, held by the examiner. The student has an identical sheet in front of him. Any word that the student reads incorrectly is struck out on the examiner's sheet, leaving correctly read words (or letters, on the K level) blank. Above the words he has failed to read correctly the examiner writes the actual pronunciation the child gave, for further analysis of errors at a later date. For example, we record

F	make	tree	cow	about
~~S~~	m~~a~~n	th~~r~~ee	thr~~o~~w	ab~~o~~ve

Analysis of errors will be helpful if remedial programming is indicated. In order for the child not to lose the line on the sheet, a plain sheet of bond paper can be placed immediately under the line being read.

For scoring the recording sheet, count the number of words read correctly, including the first line (K) up to the break-off point, which is six consecutive failures. One point is given for each word or letter read correctly on lines K through 3. For all words read correctly on lines (grades)

4, 5, and 6, give *two points*. There are 10 words to each line (grade) for K through 3, and 5 words for lines (grades) 4 through 6. The Reading Estimate form allows for a quick calculation of the total point score. The total sum of points, for example, 46, represents the raw score, which is also our final score if we place a digit in front of the last number, like this: 4.6. Our child is reading on the fourth-grade level, in the sixth month of that particular grade. This is also considered as the Reading Grade Equivalent, or his level of reading success for oral word recognition. For example, if the child read 26 words correctly, his score is 2.6, meaning second grade–six months, or halfway through the school year. If the youngster recognized only 6 letters on line K, his score is .6. If he picks up 1 word on line 1, his score is .7, even though he read 1 word on the first-grade level. After line 3, 2 *points* are given for each word read correctly, and added into the total sum of points.

It must be stressed again here that the final results represent an estimate of the child's ability to recognize words orally. We do *not* test phonetic ability or comprehension. The reason for pointing this out is that some children read at a higher level if the words are presented in context, where pictorial and contextual clues will give them hints. The fallacy of giving pictorial clues is discussed later.

B. Checklist of Characteristics of Specific Learning Disabilities

The following checklist will help teachers and parents to determine the existence of a reading problem. To a limited extent it also helps to spot spelling, writing, and arithmetic problems. There is no precise dividing line between good and poor readers for this checklist, but for a specific learning disability to be suspected, *several signs* must be present, and even then the results can only serve as a guide, in conjunction with other indicators. But this procedure is far better than mere guesswork! It is not only the total number of characteristics checked off which serves as an indicator of a learning problem; but the number, intensity, and persistence of the combined difficulties and symptoms should also give cause for concern and thus warrant further investigation and professional testing. The checklist will serve as a very good starting point by taking the child's problem out of the worrying stage into the ACTION STAGE.

CHARACTERISTIC SIGNS OF SPECIFIC LEARNING DISABILITIES

Rudolph F. Wagner, Ph.D.

General Observations

	Yes	No
1. Is the student's intelligence within the broad range of "average" or above, based on observations, group test results, comparisons, and other indications?	☐	☐
2. Does the school record indicate reading difficulties from the first grade? Do teachers' comments include statements such as "He could do it if he tried" or "He seems to have higher potential"?	☐	☐
3. Has he ever received special tutoring with conventional teaching methods for reading, but shown little or no improvement afterward?	☐	☐
4. Is his reading level two years or more below expectancy with respect to his mental ability and educational opportunities? (In children ages five to seven, this discrepancy would be less than two years.)	☐	☐
5. Does he forget previously learned words some days, but remember them on other days?	☐	☐

6. Is there evidence of similar reading difficulties in other male members of the family line? ☐ ☐
7. Does he show emotional reactions to the reading problem, such as a strong aversion to reading, feelings of inferiority, aggressive tendencies, or behavior problems? ☐ ☐
8. Does he feel "stupid," not smart, because he cannot read like others in his class? ☐ ☐
9. Were there any injuries or significant incidents before, during, or after birth? ☐ ☐
10. Has he ever been seen by a medical doctor because of hyperactivity or nervousness? ☐ ☐

Perceptual Abilities and Orientation

11. Does he have difficulties in following a series of detailed directions? Does he mix up yesterday and tomorrow? ☐ ☐
12. Is he unable to recall with reasonable accuracy a series of events in proper time sequence? ☐ ☐
13. In his reading of text, does he omit words and phrases, skip lines, or lose his place? ☐ ☐
14. Does he have difficulty in school, copying words correctly from the board? ☐ ☐
15. Does he frequently ignore parts of words, both in copying and in reading? For example, does he read "stilt" for slit, "cover" for clover, or "plot" for pilot? ☐ ☐
16. Does he often and persistently read some words from right to left, such as "was" for saw, "pot" for top, or "no" for on? ☐ ☐
17. Does he have mixed dominance, that is, does he use the eye opposite his dominant or preferred hand? Can he use both hands equally well when writing? Does he kick with the foot opposite his writing hand? ☐ ☐
18. Does he show evidence of poor orientation in space? Does he experience difficulty in telling left from right during games and activities? Are directional concepts confusing in general, for example, east and west, before and behind, days of the week? ☐ ☐

Perceptual-Motor Activities

19. Does he show poor ability to reproduce rhythm in sequence? ☐ ☐

48

20. Is his handwriting cramped, slowly done, or very messy? Does his written work show many erasures, mark-outs, or mistakes in general? Is his work poorly spaced in general, such as words too far apart or running together? ☐ ☐
21. Does he frequently miscopy a word in one place and copy it correctly in another? For example, he may spell *house* as "hous," "hose," "horse," or "hours," all on the same page of work. ☐ ☐
22. Does he often make letter and number formation from down to up or from right to left, starting at the wrong place, but perhaps ending with the correct symbol? ☐ ☐
23. Does he habitually and persistently reverse some of his letters and/or numbers? For example, *b* for *d*, *6* for *9*, *12* for *21*, or *p* for *q*? ☐ ☐
24. Is his motor coordination poor, either in using play equipment or in manipulating smaller objects in the classroom or at home? Does he hold his pencil in a clumsy way when writing? Is he considered awkward by others? Does he drop things easily? ☐ ☐
25. Does he appear clumsy when hopskipping? Does he throw a ball with his right arm but write with his left, or vice versa? ☐ ☐

Speech and Language Behavior

26. Is his speech immature, like baby talk? Was he slow in learning to talk? ☐ ☐
27. Does he sometimes confuse the order of syllables in multi-syllabic words, such as "japama" for *pajama*, "pasghetti" for *spaghetti*, and "aminals" for *animals*? ☐ ☐
28. Does he have difficulty pronouncing words that contain consonantal clusters, such as *episcopal*, *statistics*, or *crisp biscuits*? ☐ ☐
29. Does he have difficulty in hearing sound difference between similar words, such as *pin/pan*, *lease/leash*, *bend/bent*, or *his/hiss*? ☐ ☐
30. Does he show a poor ability to associate sounds with letter symbols? Or, can he give the proper sounds of letters individually while he is unable to blend the sounds into words? ☐ ☐

31. Is his comprehension of materials greatly influenced either by oral or by silent reading? That is, is there significant improvement in understanding when one or the other method is employed? □ □
32. Does he rely heavily on pictures in the book when reading? For example, he may look at the picture of a duck but read the printed word *bird* as "duck." □ □
33. Is his spelling particularly poor or even bizarre in original compositions? Does he make errors such as "cud" for *could* "luns" for *lunch*, and "wuns" for *once*? □ □
34. Did he ever develop a stutter, possibly after attempts were made to change his handedness? □ □
35. Did he have a significant delay in speech or show difficulty with certain sounds that persisted for a while, especially the *r*, *w*, and *th* sounds? □ □

C. An Inventory for Letter and Word Reversals

The purpose of the Inventory for Reversals is to help spot children who have specific reading disabilities often undetected until it is too late to remediate the problem. The Inventory is *not* an achievement test and should be used only in conjunction with other tests of a diagnostic nature. The assumption underlying the Inventory is that children with specific reading problems have greater difficulty with oral reading, and make more letter and word reversals, than children of the same age and comparable intelligence. For example, children with severe reading problems may read "buck" for *duck*, or "saw" for *was*. Reversals also occur in consonantal clusters, such as "blot" for *bolt*. By counting the reversals on a standardized inventory in an objective way rather than subjectively noticing them in a child's reading habit, it is possible to compare the results with errors children of average reading ability make at the same age. Reversals do occur in younger children also as part of a normal developmental stage.

Beyond the observation that children with reading problems have larger numbers of reversals than normal children it is further assumed that the cause of reversals in poor readers may be due to perceptual difficulties, lack of spatial orientation, and possibly underlying neurological deficiencies of a milder borderline nature. But whatever the underlying cause, reversals made by children in reading and spelling manifest themselves at what is referred to as the behavioral level, that is, the level where we can observe the reversals with our own eyes and ears. On the other hand, there are children who are poor readers—that is, their reading is below the expectancy level when age and intelligence are considered—but they do *not* show significant reversal errors in their reading or spelling. In these instances the causative factors may have to be sought in poor auditory discrimination and lack of phonetic sensitivity, among other possibilities.

Administration of the Inventory for Reversals is quickly done. The usual instructions for test-taking situations apply: good rapport should be established with the child, and no prodding or correcting must occur. The Inventory applies only to children within normal limits of intelligence (approximate IQ range from 90 to 110), or above average. It does not apply to children with special handicaps or to those who are considered mentally retarded. The child is given the Inventory Sheet (see page 58) and the examiner says to the child, "Please read these letters and words for me!" The examiner has a duplicate of the sheet in front of him to record the errors. The child is requested to read the letters and words aloud, but if he falters or hesitates for longer than half a minute, the examiner says, "Just go on to the next word!"

The Inventory does not apply to children under age 6 because many will not know their alphabet by this age if they are potentially poor readers. There are three levels on the Inventory, to be given in accordance with a child's age and attained reading ability, as follows:

Level I   Ages 6 and 7, or in cases where the child is older but cannot read whole words contained in Level II.

Level II   Ages 8 to beginning of 9 (Chronological Age 9 years but no months beyond). These children must begin at Level I.

Level III   Age 9 and up; i.e., a child is qualified for this level if he has reached the ninth year, beginning with 9 years and one month. All children in this group are started at Level I and continue with Levels II and III.

There are twenty letters and words, respectively, in each level, all intended as "traps" inviting the poor reader to reverse letters and words.

Scoring the Inventory is done while the child reads. A letter or word which is completely misread is struck out and not considered in the final count of errors. If a reversal occurs, the scorer writes the letter or word as read by the child above the words on the recording sheet and underlines it as one error. Here are some examples:

	b			b	d	d	p
Level I	<u>d</u>	m	N̸	<u>d</u>	<u>b</u>	<u>p</u>	<u>q</u>	Errors: 5

	saw	top		dip	from	no	on
Level II	<u>was</u>	<u>pot</u>	b̸at	damp	f̸or	<u>on</u>	<u>no</u>	Errors: 4

	tip	pott	slot̸	form	grat̸	boss
Level III	<u>trip</u>	<u>plot</u>	slit	<u>from</u>	<u>brag</u>	<u>sob</u>	Errors: 5

In Level III, omissions of single letters in a word are also counted as errors, but not words that are mispronounced entirely, such as "off" for *from*. It should be noted that if a child reads "d" for *p*, it also is considered a reversal error. Letters and words that the child reads correctly are left unmarked on the recording sheet. Errors may occur by left-right reversal of single letters in isolation (Level I) as well as within a word, or their *position* within the word may be reversed. For example, *b* might be read "d," *bad* as "dad," or *lap* as "pal." Up-down reversals are also counted; e.g., *n* for "u," or *M* for "W."

At the end of the reading session, the number of reversal errors is written on the appropriate line in the right-hand margin of the recording sheet. The total number of errors (sums of appropriate levels administered) is also entered at the bottom of the recording sheet. The examiner may also wish to note his observations, including dominance of eye, hand, and foot, as additional data for future evaluation.

Evaluation of the Inventory for Reversals is based on the child's age and the number of errors he made. The following norm table will serve as a guide for evaluation.

Number of Errors

Level	Age Range	Normal Reader	Border-line Reader	Problem Reader
I	6–7	0–3	4–5	6+
II	8–9	0–2	3–4	5+
III	9 up	0–1	2–3	4+

The figures above are not absolute, as is the case with any statistical data based on samples of a given population. To assist the user of the Inventory for Reversals in further evaluation of the results, the table given below might be helpful for planning a remediation program. However, no single test or inventory can serve as the basis for remedial planning or programming; the child's problem is regarded as a multiple one and should be considered on the basis of several observations and measures.

Remedial efforts for children in category B in the table should be directed toward intensive training of auditory discrimination and phonetic skills, while children in category C must be offered intensified training in left-right orientation and perceptual exercises. Resource material for the recom-

Guide for Remedial Planning

Reading Level	Reversal Errors	Category
Normal reader	No significant number of reversal errors	A. Normal reader
Below-normal reader*	No significant number of errors, or borderline	B. Possibility of difficulty with auditory discrimination and lack of phonetic sensitivity.
Below-normal reader*	Excessive number of reversal errors	C. Perceptual deficiencies may exist, with or without underlying neurological causes. Professional evaluation indicated.

* The reading level below expectancy level, i.e., poor reading, is determined by the following estimation formula: Actual Age (A) minus 6 equals Expected Reading Level (ER). For example, a child at age 12 would normally be expected to read at least at the sixth-grade level (A minus 6). It is common practice in education to consider a child a poor reader if he reads approximately 1–2 years *below* ER. However, this difference is *much less* in the early elementary grades.

mended training procedures will be found in a later chapter.

In summary: we have presented three devices which may help teachers and parents to assess their children's reading problem, after they have ascertained that the child's intelligence is at least normal, and no severe emotional disturbance or physical illness exists. The procedure is especially recommended for people living in areas where professional help is not immediately available, but action is needed to reduce anxiety and concern over the child's reading dilemma. The *ideal* situation of course calls for complete professional diagnostics and recommendation for remediation by qualified professionals. But ideal situations are as yet not the rule. The next best step is self-help, to whatever limited extent.

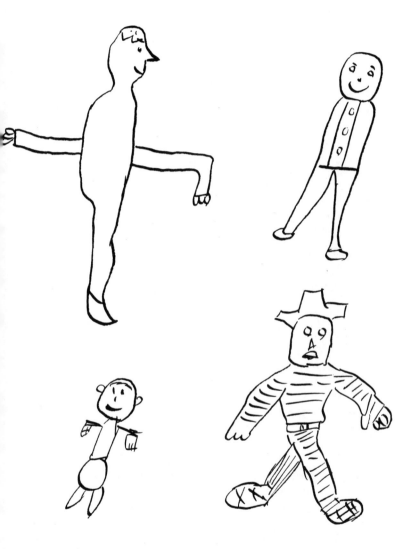

DRAWINGS BY DYSLEXIC CHILDREN. *Most children draw themselves when asked to draw a person. It is a sort of drawn self-image. Dyslexic children often see themselves handicapped and distorted, omitting details of the body and confusing spatial and size relationship. Note crippled or omitted arms, incorrect junctures, and missing eye pupils in these drawings.*

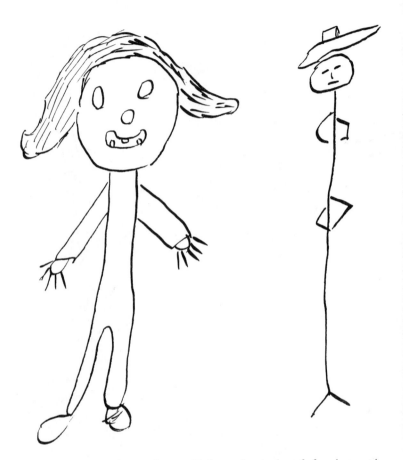

Left: Drawing by an 8-year-old boy who preferred drawing a picture of his sister. The boy is of borderline intelligence as measured by conventional tests, but this drawing shows a higher intellectual potential (note details and accuracy of some of the body features). In the classroom, he is fidgety, nervous, distractible, and a budding behavior problem. Placed in the third grade, he barely reads on the second-grade level. The mother reported difficulties during pregnancy (bleeding). His older brother likewise has a reading and spelling problem.   Right: The drawing of stick figures is often done by children with specific learning problems. This 10-year-old boy tried to cover up his inability to draw body outlines by producing a simple stick figure. Even in this attempt at oversimplification he shows inaccuracies in detail and junctures. Placed in the sixth grade, he reads on the mid-third-grade level.

Estimation of Reading Grade Level

(Oral Word Recognition Only)*

Grade Level	.1	.2	.3	.4	.5	.6	.7	.8	.9	1.0
K	O	T	C	S	F	L	K	m	h	GOOD
1	man	milk	cow	school	boy	tall	mother	look	small	woman
2	room	young	water	green	love	above	three	child	drink	dear
3	ocean	cause	stream	write	idea	strong	exact	price	throw	tongue
4	result		district		quantity		nervous		easily	
5	situation		property		severe		height		anticipate	
6	numerous		proceed		thrifty		usage		scalpel	

Name of Child: _____ Age: _____ Total Words Read (K–3, 1 pt.) _____
Total Words Read (4–6, 2 pts.) _____

Total Points: _____ Estimated Grade Level _____

* See text for instructions for administration and evaluation. Not to be reproduced in any form without permission from the publisher or author.

Inventory for Reversals
(Oral Word Recognition Only)*

LEVEL
I II III

										Number of Reversal Errors →
LEVEL I (Ages 6–7)	b	d	p	q	g	m	d	P	u	n	
	N	b	M	p	w	q	d	b	d	W	_____
LEVEL II (Ages 8–9)	was	dab	but	bib	saw	tub	bid	of	bed	top	
	for	no	dip	pot	on	dump	pad	pig	lap	bat	_____
LEVEL III (Ages 9 up)	plot	spot	tilt	blend	belt	slit	stilts	skip	blot	from	
	trip	brag	clove	quit	sobs	felt	bolt	crib	garb	pelt	_____

Name of Child: _____ Age: _____ Grade: _____ Sex: _____

Estimated Intelligence Level: Below Average / Average / Above Average

Lateral Dominance: Hand left/right; Eye left/right; Foot left/right

Total Number of Reversals: _____ (Indicate Levels Administered: I II III)

* See text for instructions for administration and evaluation. Not to be reproduced in any form without written permission from the publisher or author.

PERCEPTUAL INACCURACIES AND DISTORTIONS. *The reproductions here were drawn by dyslexic children in response to the presentation of sample figures shown in the left-hand column. All the children have at least average intelligence.*

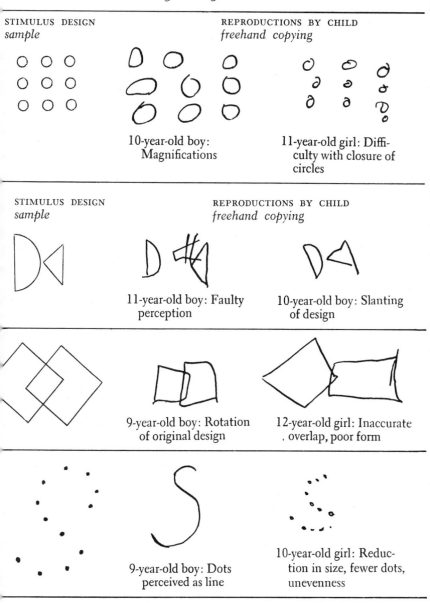

STIMULUS DESIGN
sample

REPRODUCTIONS BY CHILD
freehand copying

10-year-old boy:
Magnifications

11-year-old girl: Difficulty with closure of circles

STIMULUS DESIGN
sample

REPRODUCTIONS BY CHILD
freehand copying

11-year-old boy: Faulty perception

10-year-old boy: Slanting of design

9-year-old boy: Rotation of original design

12-year-old girl: Inaccurate overlap, poor form

9-year-old boy: Dots perceived as line

10-year-old girl: Reduction in size, fewer dots, unevenness

5 · WHERE TO GET HELP

While the basic theme of this book is one of self-help, there will come the time when a puzzled and desperate parent or teacher will have to seek professional help. This chapter lists some of the people who are professionally qualified by training and experience to offer needed counsel and advice. Parents with dyslexic children are indeed in a dilemma, since desperately searching for help can often be a very frustrating task. What if the family lives in a rural setting, away from metropolitan centers where professionals usually cluster? A reading clinic might be located miles away, sometimes hundreds of miles. And what is even more upsetting at times is the fact that after all examinations and tests have been completed and a diagnosis has been established, the parents and child are referred back to the educator, who is to follow through with the suggestions and recommendations. Parents and children who have gone through such a vicious circle will readily attest to the confusion they had to go through. Others may have been more fortunate and selected the right place and the right professionals in the first place. Being informed about the problem and what it entails can save time and money from the start. Ideally, after the diagnosis has been made, a precise recommendation for remediation and/or therapy should be dispensed to the educator—the so-called prescriptive teaching method. However, many teachers and school personnel are as yet not familiar with specific remedial techniques, and the bewildered parent will once again be at a loss as to what to do. But the ignorance that exists in some schools must not prevent the parents from seeking all the information necessary and available to establish a professional diagnosis, instead of listening to well-meant laymen's advice.

The Educators

As was pointed out in previous chapters, the teacher can be extremely helpful in detecting cases where a specific reading problem is suspected. The cumulative folder on the child in school contains valuable anecdotal information. For instance, intelligence, mental maturity, and reading achievement or readiness tests are periodically administered in most school systems across the country. The results of these tests can be used to gain insight into the child's standing compared with his classmates, the national norm, or simply children of his own age. Areas of weakness in learning sometimes also can be discerned by the alert teacher. The teacher will usually be reluctant to give out exact scores such as the Intelligence Quotient (IQ), but he will not want to deny the cooperative parent counsel as to where his child's abilities lie, that is, in the average, above-average, or below-average range. Tests are sometimes of limited reliability and validity, anyway, and caution must be exercised in putting too much emphasis on single scores. However, if these scores are expressed within broad ranges, such as average, below, or above, they not only become more meaningful to the parents, but also more confidence can be invested in them.

In addition to the classroom or homeroom teacher, there are many other school officials with whom the student comes in contact during the year once a reading problem has been reported to the principal or central administration. These teachers and officials may be found working under various labels, such as

Remedial Reading teacher	Visiting teacher
Language Arts teacher	Social worker
Reading Specialist	Pupil Adjustment worker
Reading Consultant	Resource teacher
Speech and Language teacher	Learning Disabilities teacher
Speech Therapist	LD coordinator
Teacher of the Dyslexics	Itinerant teacher
Language Specialist	

and many others. Each of these teachers may be called in to help in the remedial task of learning problems. For contacting these workers, again the classroom teacher, homeroom teacher, or school counselor may be of great help in arranging for an interview. The parents must find out what personnel is available in a given school system and must seek the advice and counsel of these people. Close contact with the teacher is one of the prime requisites of showing the school that the parents are interested in or alarmed about their child's progress in school. Listening to advice, rather than doubting or fighting, is likely to bring about the best cooperation and early help from the school.

Thus, getting the facts from the school is the first step. The long search for help might end there if the school system is well-equipped and staffed to handle a specific reading problem. If help is not forthcoming, the parents must then set out to find professional personnel in the surrounding communities.

The Specialists

Hearing and Vision

After a reading disability has been suspected or identified, the first bit of advice usually offered to the parents is to get the child's eyes examined. At this point, confusion already confronts the anxious parents. Who should be consulted first? Does the child need glasses or could his eyes be outright sick? When glasses are prescribed, the child will see better but not necessarily read better. For the information of parents and educators, the following distinctions are made regarding professionals concerned with vision:

Ophthalmologist. He is a member of the medical profession, and specializes in the examination, treatment, and surgery of eyes and eye diseases. He also tests eyes and prescribes glasses. He was formerly known as an oculist.

Optometrist. He tests eyes and prescribes glasses. Most optometrists also practice physical therapy for eyes (eye exercises), but they neither diagnose nor treat eye diseases from a medical standpoint.

Optician. He specializes in making glasses according to prescriptions. He is not an eye expert in the medical or optometric sense.

Just where to start if a visual problem is suspected may depend on many factors, but the following statement may serve as a guide: if poor eyesight is suspected, an optometrist might be consulted first. Suspicion of an actual eye disease would call for an ophthalmologist. In either case, a responsible professional specialist will make the appropriate referral to the other eye expert.

In cases where the child's hearing ability is questioned, the otologist is needed, also called an ear doctor, a medical person. He would be the professional to go to in case of hearing defects or poor listening abilities as the possible cause of poor reading. This specialist would perform an otoscopic examination or call certain technicians to run other tests, for example, an audiometric test (hearing test) or evaluation of the child's speech by a speech correctionist or therapist. Hearing, listening, and speaking are often interrelated, and difficulty in one area may cause difficulty in another. It might be that the child's hearing acuity—that is, the ability to hear sounds—is all right, but his ability to discriminate sounds is defective. The words *pin* and *pen* may sound exactly alike to him. If such defects can be identified, remedial exercises are available and very beneficial to the child's reading progress. Something *can* be done for the struggling youngster.

But the array of specialists who may help in the proper diagnosis of learning disabilities does not end here. Next we turn to more medical persons who have a central interest in the subject.

Mind and Body

Many people find it advisable to start their journey in search of their child's cure by making an appointment with their family physician. This is quite in order, since this person would not only know the family but could suggest reliable resources and medical specialists available in the community.

Neurologist. This "nerve doctor" is a member of the medical profession and specializes in the diseases of the human nervous system. He will examine a person's reactions and reflexes, investigate the medical history going back to prenatal incidents and order special tests where needed, e.g., the brain wave test or electroencephalogram. He will prescribe drugs such as tranquilizers or antidepressants if indicated. The neurosurgeon performs operations on the nervous system, including the brain.

Pediatrician. An M.D. specializing in childhood diseases or their prevention, he examines children physically and can prescribe medication. The modern pediatrician has become aware of learning problems as they relate to medical findings.

Psychiatrist. A full-fledged member of the medical profession with his specialty in conditions and diseases of the mind, he employs a variety of tests and techniques to examine a person for diagnosis and treatment. His therapeutic interventions may include psychoanalysis, drug therapy, or specialized treatments involving individuals or groups. Child psychiatrists specialize in the diagnosis and treatment of children and adolescents. He may be involved in therapeutic intervention related to emotional problems as a secondary reaction to learning problems.

It should be borne in mind that the medical specialists above often establish the diagnosis of specific learning problems by ruling out organic and emotional factors. They may at times prescribe certain drugs that aid in the remediation of learning problems by making the child more amenable to learning. Drugs may affect a child's attitude and combat his irritability, nervousness, tension or anxiety, but they are not specifically aimed at the learning skills proper, such as reading. For this reason, the medical specialists may refer the parents and child to appropriate educational clinics, learning centers, child guidance clinics, or tutorial facilities where the child can be helped through special education methods.

Another professional specialist involved in learning problems is the psychologist. The profession of psychology is relatively new in this country and is beginning to specialize also. Care must therefore be exercised to choose a psychologist who has training and experience in the area of learning problems. Most states in the United States have licensing or certification laws, and the state board may be able to refer the parent to the right person. Ordinarily, a fully trained psychologist holds a Ph.D. or in some instances an Ed.D., depending on his educational background. Some states admit psychologists with a master's degree in psychology for private practice. In local, state, and federal institutions such as schools and clinics, these laws often do not apply, and position requirements are established by the institutions themselves. The following would deal especially with educational and learning problems:

Clinical Psychologist. He deals with the examination and therapy of mentally maladjusted persons and uses psychological tests to find out what causes the problem. He also engages in therapeutic efforts to bring the individual back to mental health by using individual and group counseling techniques.

Child Psychologist. He specializes in the examination and treatment of maladjusted children and adolescents, using psychological tests and therapeutic measures.

School Psychologist. Working in educational settings, he is particularly trained in methods and procedures to help children with difficulties related to learning. He is concerned about learning problems of individual children in the school and may consult with parents, teachers, and school officials. He is qualified to administer and interpret psychological tests, and also engages in individual and group counseling.

Psychometrist. A psychological technician, he administers and scores psychological tests which help toward an objective assessment of learning problems. He is qualified to administer individual intelligence and achievement tests.

Psychologists may be found in clinics and private practice. Some college professors engage in a limited private practice and can be contacted in colleges and universities which may have guidance or counseling centers attached to the institution. Psychologists working in school settings on a full-time basis as employees of the school system usually perform their services free of charge to the children and their parents. This saves parents the expense incurred when advice is sought outside the school system. To give some rough idea of such expenses, fees for a complete psychological workup may range anywhere from $30 to $100, depending on the type of tests given and the number of contacts required. Fees charged by medical specialists may be higher, especially when extensive testing is done. These tests may include the brain wave test (EEG), laboratory tests, social histories and psychological examinations, or other special tests and examinations. For persons on welfare or covered by federal, state, and local agencies (for instance, Rehabilitation Service, Veterans Administration, etc.), these expenses may be partially or totally covered.

Since learning disabilities engender signs and symptoms in one or more areas of learning and human behavior, a "team approach" is often employed by clinics and agencies to assess and help the total child. Thus we might find a host of specialists working in clinics, agencies, or schools, all zooming in on one problem. By this multidisciplinary approach, as it is called, the various specialists contribute the specific knowledge in their own fields, attempting to untangle the puzzle a child may present to them. These centers can be found under different names in the various localities: Learning Center, Guidance Clinic, Mental Health Center, Learning Disabilities Center, Evaluation Clinic, Counseling Services, or Treatment Center. If one is at a loss just whom to contact, it is advisable to ask the classroom teacher, family physician, social worker, or related personnel for guidance. Much confusion and time can be saved by exploring the community resources thoroughly for the right kind of help. Parents should beware of "schools" without the proper reputation or accreditation, since quacks will try to find their prey wherever human misery and suffering abide. Quick and speedy "cures," cut-rate prices, or persons traveling under the cloak of paraprofessionals are certainly not the answer for diagnosing and treating dyslexic children. It takes professional skill and experience to diagnose and treat a child with severe learning problems. These specific problems cannot be remedied overnight. As yet, there are no quickie methods and techniques for severe learning problems; it takes time to help this type of child and his parents.

Who will teach your child to read? The search for special tutors and trained teachers in schools and local clinics is often very frustrating—and even more often, in vain. Many people offer advice, and some even active help. A neighbor, a retired teacher, a teen-ager next door—many have the will but do not know the way. In desperation, some parents try to tutor their own children. But can a parent help here?

Under ordinary circumstances, parental tutoring is not recommended. Parent-child relationships are naturally too close emotionally. Day-to-day living under one roof lets people take things for granted. Distractions at home are numerous: just when mother and child sit down for a lesson, the phone starts ringing, the mailman comes by, or the baby starts to cry. After a short time of tutoring, mother can't stand it any longer and begins to pressure the child or fuss at him. Results are often devastating and may end in big fights, shouts, and tears. No surgeon operates on his wife except in an emergency, and no father and mother can teach their child—with some exceptions—because of the emotional closeness the relationship involves. But until a professional tutor or learning center can be located, *your situation is an emergency!* Your children cannot wait; help must be initiated NOW!

A way to overcome this emotional closeness is limiting the tutorial sessions; another way is to share the responsibility with others who have to face similar situations. These two topics will be discussed below under the headings of The 15-Minute Session and The Block Pool.

The 15-Minute Session

One of the outstanding characteristics of children with learning disabilities is that they have a very short attention span. After ten to fifteen minutes of instruction, they have simply had enough. This is why many are considered behavior problems by their teachers. The child cannot sit still and concentrate for any protracted period of time. Why, then, go beyond his span of concentration and attention? Wouldn't it make sense to limit the sessions or switch to a different kind of activity that presents a new challenge?

Another point that should be mentioned is that teachers usually do not wish their children's parents to coach them at home on the same subject or with the same readers they use in school. Leave the teaching to them, they claim, because parents might not know what the teacher is trying to accomplish and thus may either undo what the teacher has tried to put across, or even confuse the child by teaching him in a different way. Teachers want a chance to teach their students first, in the method they intend to follow. Of course, the argument makes sense. If the rule is not followed, the child may be torn between two authorities, and utter confusion will result. And confusion is definitely a detriment to effective learning—something your child does not need.

Fifteen minutes is all the child and the parents can take, anyway. This may also apply to the tutor or teacher who spends extra time with the child in the classroom or after school. After fifteen minutes, both child and tutor need a break. It's much better to take a break then and come back for another 15-minute session. But these sessions must be held consistently, every night, seven days a week. This is the secret: consistency with a system. It does not matter who does the tutoring: father, mother, or someone else in the family. Whoever has the best disposition and the knack for tutoring should do the job. Boys often respond better to fathers, and girls to mothers; but not necessarily so. Big brothers, sisters, and neighbors are often good substitutes.

But what to teach? Teach what the child apparently does not get in school during the day. Try to give him the basic stuff rather than attempting to advance him or push him over the limits. Never mind keeping up with the class average; teach at the level where he begins to fail. Give him enough easy stuff so that he can get a taste of success again. This is important. Gradually make things more difficult for him, always going back to things he already knows, lock-step style, two forward and one back. You must build up his shattered confidence. A poor self-image is part of the poor reader's problem, the idea that he thinks he is "stupid," which he is not. Where to start instructions depends on the child's present level of functioning. This was discussed in Chapter 4, and the reader should have some idea by now just where the child stands: Nonreader, hardly knowing his alphabet? Early first grade? Late second grade? That's where we must begin.

Most children are not only academically retarded in relation to their peers' scholastic performance, but they often seem also developmentally behind. Many simply seem to mature comparatively late, for example, in talking, walking, balancing, holding a pencil or a cup, or playing outdoors. Not all poor readers have this developmental lag, but many do. They are sometimes referred to as developmental dyslexics—just another term.

For example, let's take the simple task of copying a design and see how children compare with established norms—the way an "average" child would do it. Some children can perform the task at an earlier age, and some later, of course. The illustration on the next page gives an approximate yardstick for determining a child's relative standing.[1]

These selected figures are just examples of how the average child would perform in copying these designs. The quality of performance would be still another evaluative yardstick. Why are drawings used for this purpose? They seem to be good indicators of developmental stages, as has been pointed out by many authorities. The task of copying designs is used very frequently in assessing a child's developmental stage and perceptual ability.

If a child is a nonreader or reads on kindergarten level,

[1] Age norms based on *School Readiness*, by Francis L. Ilg and Louise Bates Ames, Gesell Institute for Child Development. Published by Harper & Row, New York, 1965. Reference quoted with kind permission from the authors.

FIGURE	APPROXIMATE AGE WHEN DESIGN IS SUCCESSFULLY DRAWN	
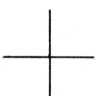	CIRCLE	Age 3
	CROSS	Age 4
	SQUARE	Age 4–5½
	TRIANGLE	Age 5–7
	COMPLEX FIGURE	Age 5½–7
	DIAMOND, FLAT	Age 7

the parent or teacher might not even attempt to coach him in reading but do simpler preparatory work, trying to develop and strengthen his perceptual powers. Suggestions for doing this are given in the next chapter. Here we only want to set the stage. The training of left-right movements is very important in this connection, since reading in our culture proceeds from left to right on the printed page. Letters like d and b are positioned in a certain way on the page, and words and sentences are read from left to right. If this left-right movement is not firmly established, reversals will result. This applies to reading as well as writing.

Many parents and teachers will be surprised at how poorly some children execute these simple exercises at first. This is precisely why they should be trained in them. There may be children who fail at a very early stage of perceptual development. If they do, we must go further down the ladder and give them even simpler exercises. Each stage has to be firmly established so that we do not build on shaky ground. We may have to draw on not just one but two or more senses to accomplish what normal children can do without crutches. If a child fails to discriminate visually between two circles of different sizes, for example, the circles could be cut out from sandpaper so that the child may trace the shapes with his dominant hand. (About 90 percent of all children are right-handed.) This is called a multisensory approach, suggested by many leaders in the field of perceptual training, among them Maria Montessori and Grace Fernald. The question of retraining the sidedness, such as left to right, will not be taken up here, since it entails more specific training procedures which, applied without thorough study of the child's behavior, might do great harm. Again, more hints and suggestions for perceptual training are given in the next chapter.

Some commercially produced material has recently come on the market, but it is relatively expensive when purchased for tutoring one individual child. Besides, the secret lies in the do-it-yourself material blended with a wholesome child-parent or child-teacher relationship. During the fifteen minutes, kindness, understanding, and calmness must prevail. Excessive pushing and constant prodding or fussing are out of place and have been tried before to no avail. The session should consist of a kind of counseling relationship saturated with warmth and empathy, focusing on academic rather than emotional problems. After all, this is the last call for reading! As the child gains in skills, the emotional by-products of his reading problem will diminish proportionately. Again it must be stressed that consistent, systematic, and continuous tutoring are important features of the fifteen-minute sessions. Nothing must disturb this setup—nothing! No excuses should be accepted, nor should any exceptions be tolerated. Rain or shine, busy or not, fifteen minutes a day!

Once the perceptual powers of the child have been strengthened through sufficient exercises in all areas, one might proceed to higher stages of learning. The transition from exercises in perception to actual reading is gradual but definitely not a "new" thing. One leads into the other. Once reading is begun, be it ever so simple and primitive, the possibilities are endless and give both parents and teachers an excellent opportunity to show their creativity and inventiveness. A good way to get started is to pick a sound (letter) or sound combination which the child has not mastered. For example, the fricative sounds s, sh, z, or ss are good ones to start with. Then come the consonant blends which are often troublesome for the dyslexic child, e.g., bl, cr, sc, or str. Since the students also have trouble with sounds, letters, and words that are easily reversed, such as distinguishing *b* from *d* or *p* from *q*, extra practice might be needed here. We must remember that these children are considered "word blind," so they have to be shown twice and treated like people who have trouble seeing and recognizing letters and words. The teaching of phonics must not be overlooked; the child must be familiar with all sounds of the alphabet. However, phonic training does have its limits. The English language is not 100 percent phonetic—70 percent at best—and thus we cannot teach English by phonics exclusively. We must supplement our phonetic training with word recognition exercises by exposing the whole word at one time and allowing the learner to become familiar with the shape and appearance of the entire word form. Each word has a distinctive configuration. One may aid the child in this form recognition by drawing a box and then asking him to fill in the letters to make the whole word. Here are some examples.

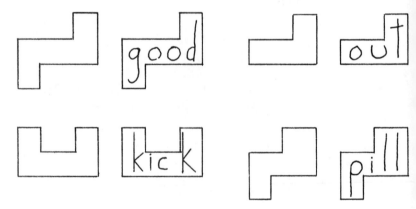

The exercise is particularly suited for children who are aphonic, that is, who have trouble distinguishing different sounds, like *pen* and *pin*, or *sip* and *zip*. This particular category of children is also referred to as auditory dyslexics —again, just another term for children who have trouble with their reading.

Another way to start the 15-minute sessions is to begin with vowels (a, e, i, o, u, and y, and combinations thereof, like ea, ay, ie, etc.). The vowels are presented in the form of phonograms—that is, words that correspond to certain rules. The short words should never be accompanied by pictures or any graphic clues, because the child will look at the pictures before he attempts to read the word, thus developing the bad habit of word guessing. Many a first grader has fooled his teacher into thinking that he can actually "read," when in fact he was guessing from pictorial clues and recalling material previously heard and committed to memory. How erroneous picture clues can be is illustrated on the drill card below.

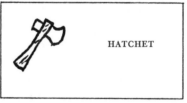

The child might read "ax," completely disregarding the word clue and responding to the picture only. Word guessers are often uncovered as late as the second grade and remediation becomes necessary, which in turn delays the child's progress.

The phonogram approach is simple and consistent. One vowel is taken up at a time, but never in isolation. The basic unit is the phonogram, which is presented by embedding it in sounds which, together with the phonogram, form a word. Nonsense words are acceptable as long as they are not overdone. To demonstrate the method, let us single out the phonogram at, as in "at the river." Here we have r-at, fat, cat, sat, mat, etc. Or let us take *it* as an example: *p-it, fit, lit, kit, sit,* etc. Or a vowel combination like *ea: p-eat, meat, feat, seat, beat, neat,* etc. The child recognizes familiar units in the word which facilitates the reading of new words. In other words, there is transfer from known to unknown words. Samples of these words may be written on small flash cards for interval checks, because dyslexic children also have trouble reading words out of context. A child may be able to read a word on a card but unable to recognize the same word on the blackboard. Practice is needed here.

The child with a severe reading problem needs both methods, phonic and word recognition, in addition to specialized training that provides the perceptual underpinning for the poor reading habits. Some children respond better to phonic training, while others cannot hear the sounds well. Feedback of success and failure in attacking new words will be the guide for choosing one method over the other. None should be employed to the extreme. Where the phonics method leaves us stranded can be shown by asking someone to sound out the word *psychology.* The initial *p* is of course not sounded because it is mysteriously silent. That's English, the system we are confronted with! Here the word recognition method must take over, even though "fonetic phanatics" would give us an ad hoc rule to prove their method: *p* before *s* is silent, *p* before *h* is not but becomes *f.* This is the reason why some teaching methods try to phoneticize the English alphabet to make it regular and consistent. But the child will still have to transfer to the conventional alphabet later on.

The Block Pool

Many parents will throw up their hands in despair if they have read up to this point. How will I be able to teach my child all of this? The suggestions and exercises, while perhaps comprehensible and sensible, are too much for some parents and teachers. This is quite an understandable reaction. There may be emotional factors which weigh against tutoring one's child. But to give up at this point would mean not responding to the last call for the child's success with reading. Abandoning the ship now will spell veritable disaster for the child and his family—educationally, culturally, personally.

Parents living in the same block or in close geographic proximity can form very intriguing collaborations. For example, one mother took her son, a poor reader, to a nearby acquaintance who had some experience with tutoring and who consented to daily sessions, while the boy's mother took her children in a group into another room in the house and read children's stories to them. Two birds were killed with one stone, as the saying goes. Some mothers have talents in arts and crafts and can impart their knowledge to children of parents whose son or daughter needs the reading sessions. Some parents may want to share a good tutor and form very small reading groups in the afternoon after school. In another instance, several parents formed a reading club and freely exchanged their children for the tutoring sessions as needed. Fathers can be helpful in making the necessary materials, such as drill cards and cutout letters. In this way, intense contact with one's own children can be minimized, and the experience of others can be shared. Many times there are volunteers, mothers whose sons and daughters have left the nest and who now find satisfaction and gratification in a tutoring job—paid or unpaid. Women's clubs are frequently interested in the subject of reading and dyslexia and can be of tremendous influence and actual help. These groups should be organized along the lines of other existing organizations, such as the "Indian Guides" of the YMCA, where fathers with their sons meet to share their relationship and skills as "Pals Forever!" Local professionals and school boards may become interested in these groups and sponsor them or provide professional consultants.

What can be done in private homes is also applicable to school situations. Parents and teachers may want to form reading clubs in their respective schools and provide the necessary impetus for success. Team teaching is a proven technique to make full use of a good reading teacher while her colleague takes over the rest of the students. Appropriate incentive programs are also very useful in keeping poor readers interested. Small tokens are given as reinforcers after a certain amount of work is mastered, and these tokens can be redeemed at the end of the day or week for something the child desires.

More "homespun" tutorial techniques for our 15-minute sessions will be presented in the next chapter. Last-ditch survival methods can be found in Chapter 12. We simply never give up on teaching our children to read. The rewards for such labor are beneficial for both parent and child.

7 · MORE EXERCISES . . .
AND THEN SOME

The normal child learns to read at the pace of one grade in one year or a 1:1 ratio. Our public schools are geared to this pace. However, the child with a learning disability will learn at a much slower pace, perhaps 1:2 or even 1:3, meaning that he will need two or three years to accomplish what the "normal" child does in one year. As the child grows older and does not benefit from conventional teaching methods, this gap becomes wider and wider. Once remediation is initiated, the child faces a dual problem: he has to catch up with his peers, but at the same time he also has to keep pace with them, since they are progressing while he is catching up—hopefully. Time is of the essence for the dyslexic child. Once we know that the child is not able to keep pace with his peers as far as reading is concerned, the race against time begins. The longer we wait with remediation, the more catching up the child has to do later. Valuable time is lost. The distinct message of this book is the importance of giving poor readers a head start on remediation. Since a full-fledged therapeutic program cannot be started until professional help and proper schools are located, here is what needs to be done in the meantime:

1. Strengthening and broadening the foundation for reading by providing the child with intensive perceptual training as needed;

2. Teaching word attack as the basic tool for accurate reading skills; and

3. Creating an atmosphere of understanding and acceptance of the child's problem to combat his weakening self-image and avoid secondary emotional reactions.

In Chapter 6 we tried to set the stage for remedial work by proposing the 15-minute session for tutor and child. Some hints as to what to do during these sessions were given. In this chapter we intend to provide the tutor with a greater variety of exercises. These exercises are only examples of what should be done and do not constitute a prescribed and programmed remedial approach. Some references for resource material of a more systematic nature are given in Chapter 8, along with names and addresses of the respective publishers or distributors.

Perceptual Development in Children

At the beginning of a child's efforts to learn how to read, he actually uses his senses more than his sense: only after the senses have picked up the symbols on the page does the child try to interpret what he has just read. Thus meaning is secondary in the beginning reading process and is actually the culmination of, or reward for, reading a text. It is probably not too difficult to see this close relationship between seeing, hearing, and other senses on the one hand, and reading on the other. In reading we use our senses first, that is, actual seeing and hearing, and then we try to interpret what we have just seen, or better, perceived. During the development of a child's perceptual ability, he goes through various predetermined stages, from primitive to more complex. If he encounters difficulty at any one stage, he falls behind, in comparison with his peers, and we consider him immature and slow in perceptual development. This developmental immaturity or maturation at a slower-than-normal pace shows up behaviorally in poorly developed perceptions and, as a consequence, in poor reading.

Since our culture is strongly oriented in the visual-perceptual realm, the world of vision receives our greatest attention, and vision becomes our primary sensory avenue to the brain and knowledge. A blind man is pretty much lost in a seeing world. Visual perception in the child starts out with the recognition of simple shapes and forms around him so that he can bring order into what looks like a chaotic environment. Until the child reaches the age of eight, developing his visual-perception abilities is one of his major developmental tasks. There are other tasks he has to learn and master along with visual perception. If the child lags behind in any one of the tasks, it is not necessary to train him in all phases of perceptual development. If he masters a task, the tutor should be cognizant of this fact and move on to the next stage in the hierarchy of tasks. However, the child should be started at a stage he has already mastered in order to gain confidence, then moved on to a more challenging exercise.

In the earlier years of remedial work with poor readers,

perceptual training, especially visual perception, was often strongly overemphasized. Children with mass-duplicated worksheets were seen busily engaged in doing their remedial work, copying designs, tracing lines, or simply filling in blanks. More recent research studies have shown that there may be no direct relationship between perceptual training and reading achievement, but perceptual training can be viewed as very worthwhile as a part of development in the hierarchical process of learning. When it is given wholesale to all children with learning problems, the positive effects are minimized and spread too thin. A child may receive exercises for visual perception, when he needs to be strengthened only in a narrow area of this modality, perhaps figure-ground relationship, or left-right discrimination. Decisions in academic therapy with children must be based on the unique *patterns* of perceptual strengths and weaknesses of an individual child. Recent federal guidelines make individualized, almost tailor-made instructions mandatory for the teacher of children in special-education settings.

The need for individualized instruction again points up the importance of a precise diagnosis, in which weak areas are pinpointed first. Next, specific programs must be planned or created to meet individual needs, based strictly upon the findings of the initial assessment. The Illinois Test of Psycholinguistic Abilities (ITPA), developed by Samuel Kirk in the 1960s, was meant to assess many of the variables that go into the reading process, even though some controversies about the test have recently arisen. Another question is also of relevance here: Should the tutor address himself to the weaknesses exclusively, which may be a time-consuming process, or call in the strengths, that is, the intact areas, to optimize the child's abilities and bring them to bear on the problem? If a child cannot get the hang of phonetics for some reason or other, should we continue to hammer phonetics intot him ad nauseam, or switch to a visually oriented word-recognition approach?

Among the various perceptual abilities, the following are particularly relevant to reading. Examples of exercises for each of the categories are given later in this chapter.

A. Visual-Motor Coordination

Visual-motor coordination is the ability to use the eyes in coordination with movements of the body or one of its parts, like the hand in writing. The smooth functioning of almost every action of the human body depends on adequate eye-motor coordination. Reading is closely allied to this coordinative ability.

B. Figure-Ground Perception

Figure-ground perception is required when the child focuses his attention on events around him. In viewing a poster design, for example, certain things stand out in the perceptual foreground while others apparently are in the background even though the design is obviously two-dimensional. In listening, the same principle applies. We can pick a certain noise or sound from among several different sounds around us, depending on where we want to focus our perceptual attention and selection. To the uninformed, the printed page is nothing but black blotches on white paper, and the child has first to develop the ability to glean the letters from the background as if they were three-dimensional. A child with perceptual difficulty in this area may appear to be inattentive and disorganized because his attention tends to jump to any stimuli that come to him first. Children with neurological handicaps are particularly affected by this phenomenon, but they can be taught through intensive training in this area.

C. Perceptual Constancy

Perceptual constancy involves recognizing an object even though the same object may change its position, so that it no longer looks exactly the same. A motor car seen from the side, front, above, or at an angle has a different shape each time it is observed, but the human brain has a remarkable mechanism of integration that lets it perceive these varying forms as one and the same thing, a car. This feature is also essential in language development in order to reduce our word power to a manageable number of essential word labels. Eskimos have more than one word for snow for this reason, because snow is important to them for their survival, and some South Sea islanders need a dozen words for coconut because the fruit looms large in their daily lives. A child with difficulty in the area of perceptual constancy may perceive a certain word in one context and be unable to recognize it in another situation or position—in a different book or on a different page, or set in different-sized type. The word GOOD is not the same as the word good. There is little if any transfer.

D. Orientation and Position in Space

Orientation and awareness of position in space are abilities to see objects in relation to oneself as the basic point of reference. To the young child, behind is always behind me, and the left side is always my left side. Some children have this reference point firmly established by the time they enter first grade, while others show a maturational lag in this area. They have not developed the awareness of position in space in reference to their own body. They have a confused, disoriented relationship to the objects around them, including printed words. Poor body awareness and body image are also reflected in their drawings of people (see illustration below). Their visual world thus becomes distorted, affecting also their ability to orient themselves in the world of the alphabet and the printed page.

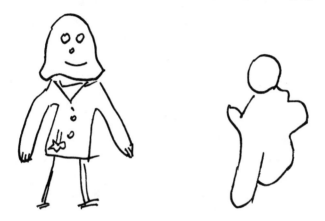

DRAWINGS BY DYSLEXIC CHILDREN *often reveal their distorted and sometimes crippled self-image by reflecting their emotional reactions to the learning disability.* Left: *An 8-year-old boy with a severe learning disability literally sees himself as a cripple.* Right: *Drawn by a 9-year-old dyslexic boy. He has no concept of his body outline and omits details. Note head dislocation.*

E. Auditory Perception

Auditory perception, or the ability to recognize sounds, is important in the reading process, since the spoken word precedes the written one. We distinguish between auditory acuity, that is, the ability to hear sounds, and auditory discrimination, the ability to differentiate between or among several sounds. Most dyslexic children are able to hear, but might have difficulty distinguishing between similar sounding words. Such inaccurate listening affects their phonetic sensitivity and they have great difficulty ascribing certain sounds to certain letters.

F. Rhythm

Rhythm seems to be a basic ingredient in reading. The term refers here to smooth eye movements from left to right on the printed page. Some poor readers show pronounced arhythmic traits in their reading. Others do not realize that a certain linguistic structure underlies sentences, with spaces for words and spaces for pauses. The same arhythmic defect can show up in speech, where it is called stuttering and cluttering.

G. Touch, Taste, and Smell

While not considered primary senses involved in reading, touch, taste, and smell are of particular concern to the poor reader, who must be reached via all possible sensory avenues, since his visual-auditory perception might be impaired. Thus, not only does strengthening of the visual and auditory senses become a prime concern to the teacher, but the effective use of other senses will aid the child in minimizing his handicap and maximizing his available sensorial resources. This is also referred to as a multisensory approach to teaching reading, and the approach is incorporated in many remedial techniques and methods. Touch, taste, and smell as senses are also known under the term *haptic system*.

The practice and exercise categories which follow will correspond to the perceptual abilities described above.

Activities for Developing Perceptual Abilities

A. Visual-Motor Coordination

GROSS MOTOR EXERCISES

Balancing:

Stand on tiptoe for ten or fifteen seconds, first with both feet, then with only one foot. Try with eyes open first, then closed.

Walk on a walking beam (an old fence, tree trunk, or beam approximately 2 by 4 inches wide and 9 feet long). Walk forward, backward, sideways. Eyes open first, then closed. Jump lightly in rhythm, do turns, anything that is safe.

Walk a chalked or taped line on the floor or on the yard. How many steps are needed to reach the end of the line? Now try with eyes closed.

Stand on one foot. How long can you stand like this? On which foot can you stand longer?

Locomotion:

Instead of walking a chalk line, crawl it: first forward, then backward and sideways, with eyes open and closed. Watch crawling rhythm and pattern; give assistance if needed.

Hop or skip on one or both feet. Watch which foot is preferred by the child. Preferred foot should be the same as dominant hand, if possible.

Imitate certain actions of tradesmen or other people, like threading a needle, dancing, drumming, ladder climbing, rowing, boxing, etc. Watch coordination; correct if needed.

Use creativity to make up new activities: marching, trombone playing, rope climbing, baseball playing, others.

FINE MOTOR COORDINATION

Cutting:

Motion with two fingers or use actual scissors; cut straight line, angles, circles, paper dolls, snowflakes, etc. For more advanced children: cut out letters of the alphabet, make small road signs, price tags, labels, and many other objects.

Placing and pasting:

Cut out certain shapes, two or three of each kind, mix them up, and ask child to match them. Felt material is very suitable, but paper will do. Vary shapes and their places on a tabletop or sheet of paper. Make shapes progressively more difficult, like hexagons, similar figures that cannot be distinguished too easily, etc.

Tracing and coloring:

Geometric figures are cut out or drawn on a posterboard or blackboard. Child traces outline in rhythm. Erase figures and see how many shapes and colors the child can remember and draw again. After work at board is successful, confine child in chair or seat and do similar exercises. Strengthen visual memory through recall of figures, shapes, and, later, letters or numbers. Watch eye-hand coordination where indicated.

Other helpful activities:

Give child opportunity to zip, button, hammer, saw, lace shoes, tie knots, do origami figures, etc.

Note: Not all children need to go through these exercises. If they have already mastered them, there is no need for overlearning. Try to establish a baseline and work up from there, increasing the complexity of the activities and exercises. Try to adapt the activities to the child's needs and age level.

MORE EXERCISES

These exercises strengthen fine motor coordination and left-right movement on a page. Increase complexity as child gains proficiency.

Put a stem on all these pretty flowers (balloons, lollipops, etc.).

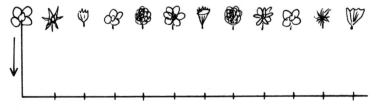

Trace the dotted line where the cat wants to get to the fish.

Complete the fence pattern around the house.

Note: The parent or teacher preparing these exercises need not be artistic. Pencil and paper are all that are needed. Children having problems with a pencil may first try crayons and old newspaper.

B. Figure-Ground Perception

DISCRIMINATING OBJECTS

Ask the child to look around in the room or outdoors, letting him name different kinds of objects that have a certain similarity. For example, show all things which are round, square, triangular, blue, pink, long and thin, horizontal, vertical, etc. Where are things that are rough when touched, soft, curved, or wet?

SORTING OBJECTS

Assemble various objects of different shapes, colors, sizes, material, texture, etc. Ask child to sort the objects according to certain categories (shapes, color, texture, material, etc.). Increase the number of categories to make task more difficult. Ask child also to classify and categorize objects around him, in the room, on the street, in the backyard.

MORE EXERCISES

Trace all the circles, squares, or other shapes, using a different color for each shape.

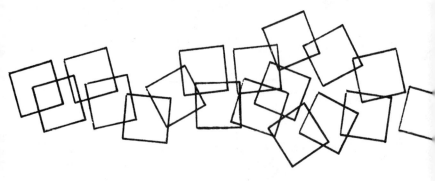

Color the shapes in No. 2 which you also see in No. 1. Compare carefully.

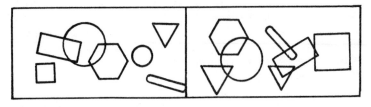

No. 1   No. 2

Trace the paths of the people and animals in the drawing. Where are they going?

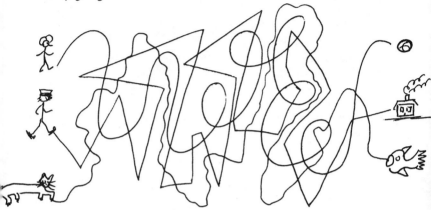

C. Perceptual Constancy

FINDING THE SAME SIZE

Give the child an object to hold, such as a colored stick, a disc or a ball. Place other objects of the same shape, but in a variety of sizes, around the child in various distances. Some of the objects should be the same size as that which the child has in his hand. The task is to identify the objects of the same size, i.e., develop good judgment for sameness or constancy.

SORTING ACCORDING TO SIZE

Cut out various shapes (circles, squares, triangles, others), using construction paper of different colors. Have several sizes of the same shapes. Now ask the child to point to the largest and the smallest shape in each variety, and then to sort them according to size, from smallest to largest.

FINDING THE SAME SHAPE

Give the child a basic design or geometric figure to start out, like a square, a triangle, or later more difficult designs. Now ask him to find like shapes in the room of any size but the same shape as the sample in his hand. For example, he may point to the tabletop for a square, or a lamp for a rod shape.

TRANSLATING DIMENSIONS

Place various objects in front of the child; then ask him to copy them on a sheet of paper, in two dimensions. Objects such as blocks, balls, tables, chairs, bridges, beds and other toys can be used for this purpose. Reproductions should be simple but accurate. The purpose is to show the child perceptual translation from three to two dimensions for the same object.

MORE EXERCISES

No. 1 is a square. Color all the squares in No. 2, regardless of their size.

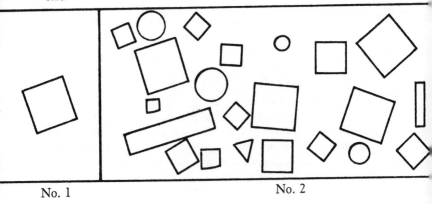

No. 1 No. 2

Here are three types of shapes. Color all circles red.

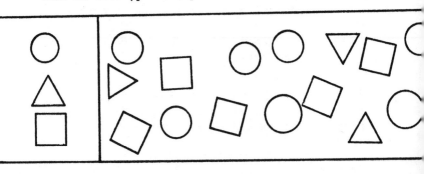

Triangle No. 1 is blue; Triangle No. 2 is red. Color all triangles of the same size according to the color samples given.

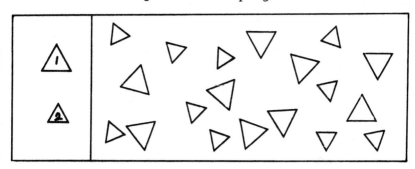

D. Orientation and Position in Space

Exercises in this category should proceed from gross to fine motor movements, and from simple to complex in task difficulty, always in accordance with the child's problem and relative proficiency. One might begin by using large objects, such as two balls, and asking the child to place a red ball in front of a green ball, or a blue cup behind, next to, or in front of a white cup. It is important that the child speak while he is doing the exercises, i.e., say "behind," "in front of," "to the left," etc., as he moves the objects.

Pegboard patterns are very helpful. Make a design with pegs or golf tees (for easy handling); then ask child to copy the design. Vary designs using different patterns and colors. Example:

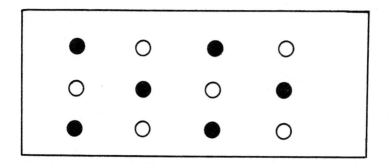

96

Complete the design of beads on a string.

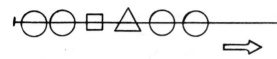

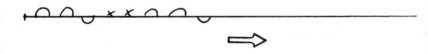

Complete the pattern.

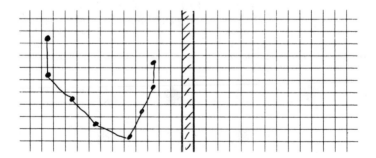

FURTHER EXERCISES WITH PATTERNS

After the child has mastered. pattern making with the pegboard, the next step is to do similar exercises, using paper and pencil. These should be done on squared paper, available in dime and stationery stores. The first designs are simple and in black pencil; later on, as the child progresses, more complex patterns and color can be introduced. The sample design is made on the left side of the paper, and the child is asked to copy the design on the right side. Examples:

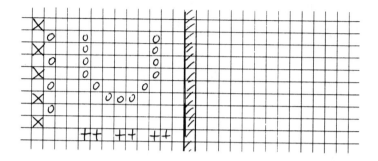

Instead of using readily available graph paper, special grid-type forms may be developed, as shown on the following pages. The first design is more basic, while the second one is for advanced work. The idea behind this exercise is that learning-disabled children with visual-perceptual problems have difficulty orienting themselves in space: life-space and paper-space. Many of these children do not know where to start, up or down, left or right, and place their beginning drawings almost anywhere on the page, without any customary sense of orientation. The exercises will give them this sense of orientation and direction by *structuring* the space for them. To go from somewhere to somewhere, you have to hop from dot to dot, thus establishing a pattern with intermittent clues.

The tutor or parent first draws simple designs on the sheet, to be followed by more complex designs as the child gains in proficiency. When errors occur, they are corrected by showing the child *how* to do it. Harsh criticism must be avoided. The atmosphere should be one of pleasant, gamelike happiness. The child might be required to trace the design first with his finger before attempting to use a pencil. Crayons might be too crude to teach this type of perceptual task. After the child has completed the design correctly but has needed several attempts to arrive at this correct trial, he may be asked to trace it with different-colored pencils, for reinforcement.

PAPER FORM BOARD

(Basic Design)

PAPER FORM BOARD FOR VISUAL-PERCEPTUAL EXERCISES
(Advanced Design)

. . . .
. . . .
. . . .
. . . .
. . . .
. . . .
. . . .
. . . .
. . . .
. . . .
. . . .
. . . .
. . . .
. . . .
. . . .
. . . .
. . . .
. . . .
. . . .
. . . .
. . . .
. . . .
. . . .

Note: When explaining or demonstrating left-right orientation exercises, the teacher should try to stand at the side of the child, in line with his vision; never in front of him. Children who have difficulty with left-right orientation in space already have a hard time doing these exercises accurately; thus any translation of 180 degrees (rotations) necessitated by the teacher's standing in front of the child would make the task much more complex for him.

Songs:

Some of the old-time standbys for learning left and right are songs like "Hokey-Pokey" or games like "Simple Simon Says . . ." where directions for movements and activities are given by the caller. Other songs suitable for this purpose are

"Looby-Loo" (*The American Singer*. Book I. New York: American Book Company, 1954, p. 97.)
"Bow, Bow, O Belinda" (*This Is Music*. Book I. Boston: Allyn and Bacon, 1962, p. 54.)

Body clues:

A child's preferred (dominant) hand may be marked with nontoxic crayon to give him a ready body orientation at all times and in all positions relative to his environment. Another way of giving such body orientation as a physical reference point is birthmarks, provided they are visible and on the dominant side.

Extraneous clues:

Special reading assignments in books may be marked as follows: Draw a GREEN circle in the left column of the page in front of each printed line or paragraph, and a RED circle in the right column opposite the green circles. GREEN stands for GO! RED stands for STOP! Observe the child's eye movements unobtrusively to check left-right ocular movements.

Paper and pencil exercises:

A large sheet of paper is placed in front of the child, such as old newspaper. The child is asked to draw lines or patterns on the sheet, always from left to right. Different colored pencils can be used to add variety. Straight lines may alternate with wavy lines or different symbols. Repeated brief exercises of this type are better than long drawn-out sessions.

Games children play:

1. *Shoot the Cannon!* Draw a small cannon on the left side of a sheet of paper. In the right margin, write a column of words which the child is able to recognize. Then say, "Shoot the cannon!" The child puts the pencil point to the mouth of the cannon and draws a line to the word which the teacher says, like "Shoot the word *apple!*" or, "Shoot *chair!*" The game ends when all words are shot, but if the child had difficulty with this series of words, the game may be repeated using a different colored pencil. Example:

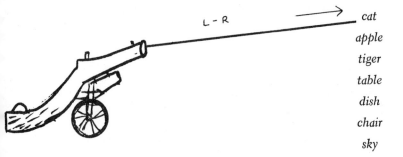

L - R

cat

apple

tiger

table

dish

chair

sky

2. *Hang the Laundry.* This is an activity for indoors and outdoors, adaptable for individuals or groups. When the title is changed from "Hang the Laundry!" to "Send a Message!" the boys will like it, too. Equipment: a laundry line or rope, sheets of paper or colored construction paper, laundry pins, crayons. The child sends out words or brief messages by writing individual letters on sheets which are hung on the line with pins, from left to right. Longer messages can also be sent out by writing whole words on a single sheet and then assembling the sentence on the line, from left to right. If there are two or more children, questions and answers can be exchanged.

3. *Calling Out Directions.* The parent or tutor gives directions to the child or group. If the direction is carried out successfully, a small prize may be earned. The directions should be made increasingly more difficult but must start at a level where the child is comfortable. If help is given, the helper must stand next to the

child, *not* facing the child but by his side. Here are examples of directions:

Touch your nose with your right hand.
Put your right hand on your left ear.
Touch your left foot with your right thumb.
Place your left foot on your right foot.
Walk two steps to the left, three to the right.
Take two steps to the left while raising your right arm.

4. *Doing the Twist.* Two or three double sheets of ordinary newspaper are placed on the floor, held together by adhesive tape to make a super-size sheet of paper. The child is then asked to lie down on the sheet, face up, and someone draws his body outline on the paper. If more than one child is available, they can take turns doing this. Eyes, ears, mouth, and other details are drawn into the figure on the paper. After this, someone gives directions to the child, like, "Put your right hand on the left ear" (of the drawn figure), or, "Can you touch the nose with your left hand, and the right toe of the left foot with your left hand?" If several children participate in the activity, they remain still while the others do their thing. The result will be a twisted scramble, and the game starts again. Directions like "Face up!" or "Face down!" may be added to make the activities more difficult.

5. *Road Maps.* A road map of any topography can be obtained readily from a nearby service station. The child is given a crayon or felt tip writer and is asked to follow directions carefully as they are given by the parent, teacher, or leader. For instance, the leader might say "Drive down Broadstreet, going west, starting at 10th Street!" After completion of the task, he may continue, "Now turn left at the third intersection!" then "Turn right at Main Street!" etc. The child traces the route with a pencil as the directions are called to him. The task does not come easily for children with orientation difficulties, so the exercises should start at a point where the child can succeed, gradually increasing in complexity.

6. *Writing on Back.* An effective way to train left-right orientation in space is to write on a child's back. The tutor writes a simple letter or word on the child's back, using his finger as a pencil and the youngster's back as the paper. The tutor stands behind the child,

both looking forward. Children who reverse simple letters, such as
d and *b*, are given practice in this area. When more complex reversals
occur in the child's reading or writing, some of these words are
used for the back-writing (for example, *was, saw, but, tub, dab, bad,*
and so on). The same method is also employed when the reversals
are mirror images, as in R and Я .

If for some reason it is not convenient to write on the child's back,
other skin surfaces can be used, such as the palm of the hand, the
arms, or even the legs. The child should have his eyes closed to take
full advantage of tactile and proprioceptive (muscular) clues.

E. Auditory Perception

AUDITORY AWARENESS AND RECOGNITION
Have child hide his eyes. Make various sounds in the room and ask
child to identify them. For example: ring a bell, tap on the table,
clink two glasses, stomp on the floor, knock at the door, etc.

Use a cheap xylophone, a piano, or several glasses or bottles filled
with different amounts of water. Train child in discriminating
between high and low tones. Tap a glass while child has his eyes
turned away, then ask him to point to the glass that was sounded.
This exercise trains both hearing (listening) and discrimination.

Ask the child to listen to the radio. Which words did the an-
nouncer say loudest, and why? Softest, and why?

Stand behind child. Say a series of words, each one softer and
softer. Determine loudness threshold when the child cannot respond any longer. Determine threshold for both ears. If in doubt
about the child's hearing, consult the school or a professional
person.

Hide a ticking clock somewhere in the room. Ask the child to find
it. Make the hiding places more and more difficult to locate.

Teach the child to sing "Old McDonald Had a Farm." The sounds
animals make are particularly appealing to the younger set.

Ask the child to identify and verbally describe sounds heard in the
house, outdoors, or in the room. Watch ticking? Refrigerator humming? A horn sounding outside?

Ask child to close his eyes. Make various sounds, like crushing paper, scratching paper, brushing carpet, etc. Ask child to identify and describe the sounds.

Note: Some of these activities are typically carried out in classes for 5- or 6-year-olds. However, many dyslexic children do not even perform on these levels and desperately need remedial work in many of the perceptual areas outlined here. Some of the exercises may have to be adapted for older children in order to keep motivation high.

AUDITORY DISCRIMINATION

Beat on drum or desk in a certain rhythmical pattern. Ask child to beat out same rhythm on his tabletop or desk. Move from simple to more complex patterns, including change of loudness, spacing, and speed.

Blindfold child and ask him to identify noises and sounds. Car going by? Someone's voice? Refrigerator humming? Radio going in adjacent room? Create your own sounds.

Record various voice samples on a tape recorder. Ask the child to identify the voices. Is the voice high or low? Does it belong to a man, woman, boy, or girl? Does he know their names? In the same manner, record various sound effects and ask child to identify them. (Running water, paper being crumpled, a knock at the door, etc.) Say two words which sound almost alike—*ball* and *fall*, or *pot* and *pet*. Ask the child if the two words sound alike or different. Increase difficulty gradually, making differences smaller or adding more words to the series. Which word in this triad sounds different: fat—fat—fit?

Fill several glasses with different amounts of water. Ask the child to arrange the glasses in order of tone level (low–high), starting at his LEFT and moving to the right. Use empty pop bottles for the same task; increase complexity by adding more bottles.

AUDITORY MEMORY AND RECALL

Play the game "Simon Says . . ." by asking the child to respond to the directions of the caller. Increase the directions in length and complexity.

Ask the child to write down from memory: first letter in the alphabet; third letter in his last name; last letter in the word *hope*; etc.

Give directions to the child, increasing memory span gradually as he attains more competence and confidence. For example: Take this pencil and put it on this chair. Go to the table, get book and put it on the chair. Open the door, touch the radio, then come back and close the door behind you, sit in club chair, fold hands.

Have child repeat commands orally before he proceeds with carrying out directions.

Increase the child's memory span by naming objects you want to buy in a store. For example, say, "I went to a grocery store and bought—3 apples, 5 bananas, one pound of coffee, cereal, a jar of pickles," etc. Have child repeat the entire series of words. Child must reach success before proceeding to more complex series.

Show the child a picture. Name several things you see; then ask child to repeat the things you saw together, but remove the picture from sight. How many things did he remember? Was he distracted? Did he respond to picture clues or the names you pronounced?

Older students may increase their memory span by having a person read words or phrases out of a textbook, to be repeated in proper order by the student. For example: *cell—nucleus—protoplasm—wall—bodies—etc.*

Choose a multisyllabic word, but do not pronounce it entirely. Leave out parts of it—at the beginning, middle, or end. For example: Safet——; ——struction; be——ning; te——phone. The same exercises can be done in visual perception where the child must complete words with missing parts.

How many things (words) can the child recall within one minute? For instance, words beginning with *s*? Words ending in *ing*? Words that start with *ch*? Etc.

MORE EXERCISES

Put an X on the picture that starts with the same sound as at the beginning of the word *hippie*.

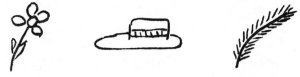

Which picture rhymes with *fat*? Put an X on it.

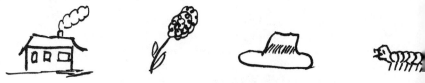

Put an X on the picture that *ends* with the same sound as in the word *fat*.

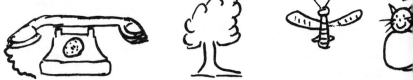

These are merely examples of things that need to be done with children who have difficulty in perception. Some children may have difficulties in one area, such as the visual, while not in others. Younger children are more likely to have these difficulties, but in severe cases of reading problems older children may have trouble as well. There are still other cases of reading problems where the perceptual areas are relatively normal but other abilities are affected. Beyond this, a child may have developed such strong secondary emotional reactions to his primary problem (i.e., reading) that he will resist this particular type of basic training in perceptual ability. By making the exercises as appealing as possible, along with wise counseling and coaching, a child may yield to this strategy sooner or later.

The following exercises in auditory discrimination and rhythm are for cases where the child may have a particularly undeveloped sense ability for audiovisual integration (connecting sound with written symbols) and basic rhythm as applied to reading. Finally, some aspects of the multisensory approach to teaching reading are discussed.

TRANSLATING AUDITORY SIGNALS INTO VISUAL SYMBOLS

Auditory discrimination requires, among other things, that the child correctly recognize and interpret auditorily perceived signals, be these beeps sent from a satellite or words in a book. In connection with reading, these signals have to be translated into written symbols, whether these are dashes and dots as in the Morse Code or words made up of an alphabet. When a word is dictated to the learner, he receives the message with his ears and writes it down using eye-hand coordination. Vice versa, if he picks up the written symbols through his eyes or visual perception and then speaks these symbols by translating them into sound patterns, he is doing oral reading. A child with reading difficulties needs training in both directions, and the following equipment will aid in this endeavor.

First, a "machine" is built which transmits signals. A simple telegraph key hooked to a buzzer or bell and a battery is constructed by mounting these parts on a board, as shown in the sketch on the next page:

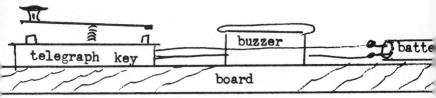

telegraph key   buzzer   batte

board

Second, a set of three-by-four-inch cards, procured from any dime or stationery store, is prepared by writing symbols on them. These symbols look like Morse Code but represent patterns of dots and dashes in a random order, ranging from simple to more complex patterns. A signal board and a set of cards are also available commercially, but they are made quickly and much less expensively by the do-it-yourselfer. Here are two sample cards:

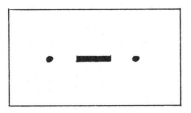
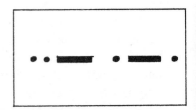

Third, the tutor is ready now to expose the cards, one at a time, and ask the student to beep out the symbols by translating them into auditory signals—that is, dashes are long beeps and dots are short beeps. The tutor can correct any mistakes the student may make, either verbally or by beeping out the symbols himself as an example.

Using the same apparatus and set of cards, the exercise can be done in reverse. The tutor beeps out a signal pattern, and the student is asked to select the correct visual pattern from a set of three to four cards placed in front of him. For example, the tutor may beep out LONG—LONG—SHORT, and the student then selects the card which has the symbol pattern DASH—DASH—DOT.

The exercise in auditory training and visual discrimination with the telegraph key goes much beyond strengthening the child's listening skills to involve the touch sense and visual recognition and discrimination, all essential features of the reading process.

F. Rhythm

USE OF THE TYPEWRITER

Many devices and gadgets have been offered in the past to help the dyslexic and dysgraphic child overcome his handicap. Usually, but not necessarily always, a child may be not only a poor reader but also a poor speller and have difficulty with his handwriting. Especially where mild neurological impairments are known to exist, the child's handwriting is shaky, messy, and often illegible, in addition to showing jumbled letters and poor orthography. Someone even suggested teaching these children Braille, considering their handicap equal to blindness. However, in the author's opinion, this method would provide a bad crutch for them and would condemn them forever to the dark world of the blind.

The typewriter has been tried as a substitute for poor handwriting and can conceivably be used during brief exercises of spelling which would have a transfer to better reading. Certainly the rhythmical element is useful in addition to avoiding writing by hand, often a slow and painful task for the small child. He may either copy spelling words or sentences from a reader, or words may be dictated by the tutor. Attention must be given to the systematic introduction of sounds and their corresponding letter symbols, from simple to complex. The children will have great difficulty, especially with the consonant blends, such as *plot*, *scramble*, or *catch*, where several consonants are bunched together. It becomes even more difficult a task in words like *Episcopal*, *statistics*, or *arithmetic*. Here is how a girl wrote a message to her mother:

> Daer mohter:
>   Paelse com home soon!
>   I need hepl wiht pselling.
>   Love,
>   Caorline

The use of the typewriter as a remedial technique can be improved upon by covering up all letter symbols on the typewriter keyboard, introducing the letters one by one by location and touch, thus excluding the faulty visual perception of these children. But the procedure is more cumbersome and requires more time to learn using the typewriter. The approach is similar to the touch system. It also avoids hand dominance.

G. Touch, Taste, and Smell Discrimination

Touch, taste, and smell discrimination can be developed through the child's food experiences. For those children whose experiences have been limited, activities should be provided to give them these experiences. The experience per se must be coupled with expressing oneself in words, and as a further step, the words should be read, and finally, written. For example, a child may smell an orange while blindfolded, say the word *orange*, and later read the word *orange* in proper context. Touch is used early by the child when he begins to explore his environment through curiosity. The small infant uses the touch sense frequently and later will be able to recognize shapes and sizes. Blind children rely almost exclusively on this sense for their type of "reading." Children with reading difficulties need this extra sense to fortify their audiovisual approach to reading. It bolsters their deficient sensory avenues and compensates for certain weaknesses. The following exercises help in developing the senses of touch (kinesthetic), taste, and smell.

Put objects of various shapes in a brown bag. Name the object and ask the child to pull it out of the bag. Another version is to ask the child to feel the objects and guess their names; if he guesses correctly, he is allowed to pull the object out of the bag. Children may play this game without supervision.

Blindfold a child and place various materials and objects in front of him. He may be asked to feel sandpaper, satin, fur, wood, rough paper, etc. Correct answers may be reinforced with tokens which can be exchanged for small trinkets.

Take a sheet of cardboard paper (construction paper) and cut out various shapes, like a jigsaw puzzle. Ask the child to put it together again, first untimed, then timed. Let him race against his previous record. If thick material is used for the puzzles, the child may want to attempt putting it together blindfolded. As usual, puzzles should be simple first, then more complex, to increase the child's ability.

Maps can be cut into various pieces, following natural geographic borders (states, for example). Aid might be given to some children who have difficulty with this task by marking the correct position of the pieces, using green dots on the left side of the piece for correct placement. See illustration, page 116.

Flat objects and templates may be used by the child in tracing outlines, first with eyes open, then blindfolded. Ask child to trace objects and shapes with various colored pencils. See illustration showing inexpensive templates available commercially, page 115.

Tie a string to a doorknob or other location in the room or outdoors, unravel it to a certain distance from the object, and ask the child "to find his way home." Child is blindfolded when doing this task.

Walking beams, rails, fences, etc., is an excellent exercise to develop balance. As child gains in proficiency and agility, he may be blindfolded. Shoes should be taken off for a better grip on the beam. Safety precautions may be necessary.

Spread a thin layer of talcum powder on a desk or table in front of the child. Call out various letters and short words and ask him to write them on the table, blindfolded, to get the "feeling" for the letter or word. He must say the letter or word out loud while moving his arm. Do not drag out the exercise; five minutes per day is sufficient to maintain and sustain interest.

Prepare a series of small bottles or old jars by filling them with all sorts of aromatic substances: lemon juice, vinegar, chocolate powder, instant coffee, grape juice, celery salt, onions, etc. Label the jars with consecutive numbers and ask the child to take a whiff. On a separate sheet of paper, write the numbers in a column with the name of the smelling samples, e.g.: (1) lemon, (2) orange, (3) vinegar, etc. After each whiff the child is asked to locate the corresponding word for the substance on the sheet of paper by placing a check mark in front of the correctly identified item. Children may play this game by themselves.

The above game can be played by using things the children can actually taste, then identify by words. It is a Tasting Party.

If a child has difficulty with correct position of letters, such as b and d, or p and q, these letters can be cut out from sandpaper and glued on dark backgrounds. The child is then asked to trace the letters with his dominant hand, saying the sounds of the letters as he traces them. The task can be accomplished with eyes open or blindfolded.

Last but not least, a tutor must be creative enough to invent new exercises or improve on old ones. The tutor is not expected to be an artist or a singer or a professional inventor—but just plain resourceful.

Exactly where to start a child with perceptual exercises depends on his stage of present functioning. Age is not a helpful guide here, since the child with learning problems performs below expectancy for a given age group. An experienced teacher knows how to find a given child's level of functioning by giving him various simple tasks and moving on up to more complex ones, until the child's instructional level is found. There are commercially produced tests on the market now, but the mission of this book is one of advocating self-help, until a more precise assessment can be made. When a child experiences difficulty with a certain task level, the tutor should give occasional exercises which were done previously so that the child does not lose interest. Routine tasks must be limited in time because the child might fall asleep right in front of them, with both eyes open. These children have already faced and suffered boredom when they received training with conventional methods in the regular classroom; such mistakes must not be repeated. One or several very brief sessions per night are preferred over drawn-out sessions with tired and nervous adults. Joy of accomplishment must crown these sessions, not fussing, upset, and tears.

There are many more ways of remediating a child's poor reading performance. Some references for professional and commercially produced tests and teaching methods will be found in the selected bibliography at the back of this book.

The following chapter will give a glimpse into the variety of teaching methods of a more specialized nature. These special techniques can be used either with individual children or small groups. The following chapter also gives hints and explanations on how to do "your own thing," often the best method available.

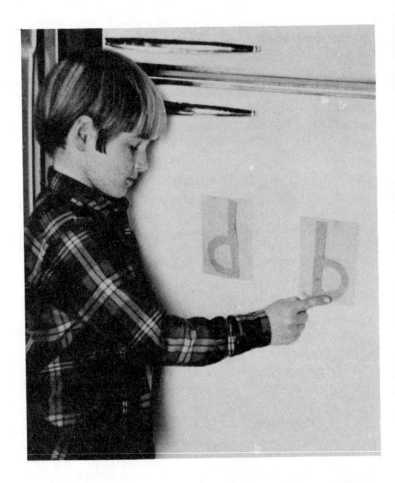

This boy, a second grader, is being helped with his reversal of b
and d by having to trace the two letters cut out of sandpaper and
attached to the refrigerator door in his mother's kitchen. To open
the door, the magic formula has to be said ("b and d") by tracing
the letters with a finger of his dominant (right) hand at the same
time.

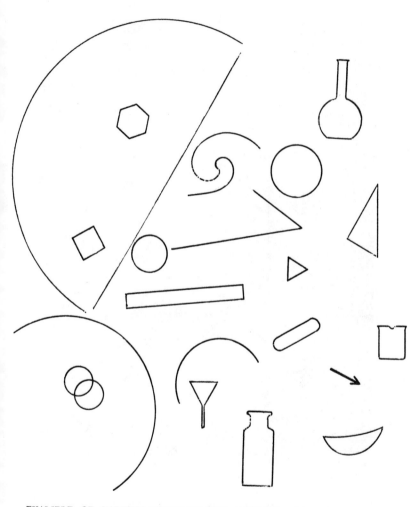

EXAMPLE OF VARIETY OF TEMPLATES AVAILABLE COMMERCIALLY. *The tracing of basic shapes and outlines is a good exercise for children with learning disabilities and perceptual difficulties. Their stroke is guided through the tactile sense until more competence is established.*

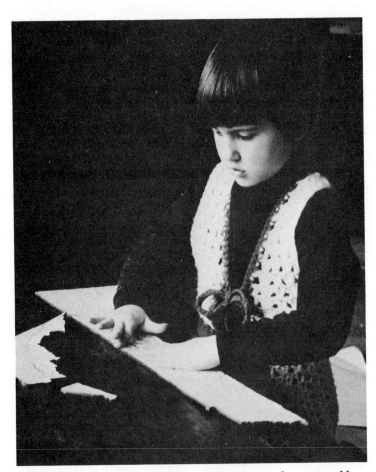

PERCEPTUAL EXERCISES. *Children with perceptual-motor problems benefit greatly from playlike exercises such as jigsaw puzzles. This young girl tries to put the shape of a state together. The puzzle is homemade, using a map readily available at a gas station and mounted on cardboard for better manipulation. Depending on the child's level of competence, these puzzles should be simple and should follow the natural contours of the picture or map. Gradually the complexity of the puzzle can be increased as the child progresses in proficiency and skill. Such exercises develop visual-motor coordination, form awareness, and dexterity—all important aspects in the reading process.*

8 · SOME SPECIFIC REMEDIAL TECHNIQUES

Most educators and parents are familiar with the two basic approaches to teaching reading in our schools today: the phonetic, or sound, method, and the whole word recognition, or "Look and say," method. Some schools use a combined approach to give the child the benefit of both methods. Not everybody, however, is aware of the fact that there are other specific techniques and methods available to teach the child who apparently has not been able to benefit from the conventional methods of teaching reading. In fact, this inability to take full advantage of the conventionally used methods of reading is one of the characteristics of the dyslexic child. If he had been able to learn how to read like others in his class, he would not be labeled dyslexic now. Before describing briefly some of the more widely known and used specific methods, perhaps a tried-and-proven, homemade approach to remediation of reading failures should be mentioned.

Depending on the child's present level of reading in respect to his expected level, a very *systematic* approach must be employed now. If the tutor goes through the phonetic alphabet with the child, the sounds must be introduced one by one. If the child has no trouble with a particular sound, the next one can be tackled without much practice. Soon tutor and child will find where intensive training is needed; usually the consonant blends give the most trouble. Difficulties with vowels are not quite so frequent. Dyslexic children have particular trouble with combining letters to form a whole word, the integrative process in reading. Here are several ways to facilitate integration of single sounds into whole words:

The phonogram technique, a linguistic approach, builds on familiar and usually meaningful letter combinations, such as *it, at,* or *car* and expands the child's word repertoire by adding single letters and letter combinations to form new words. Essentially, a phonogram is a sound made by a vowel followed by one or more consonants (e.g., *en, at, ing, old, ight*). Examples:

f → it	car ← d	r → ight
p → it	s → car	f → ight
k → it	car → ton	l → ight

The morphogram technique concerns itself with the structural aspects of the language and is best employed after the child has attained some proficiency in reading beyond the use of monosyllabic words. Here the various structural parts of a word—prefix; affix; suffix; or beginning, middle, and end positions—are used to integrate the entire word.

This is a word recognition approach basically. Example:

con — struc — tion
de — struc — tion
re — struc — ture
in — struc — tor

The various morphograms may be written on small cards and the child can form various combinations to make new words.

The flashcard approach may combine the two techniques above. The tutor writes certain words under study on three-by-four-inch cards, giving hints and explanations as needed by the reader. If a word card is recognized, it is put aside for a while, then reintroduced to make sure the reader fully masters the word, and ultimately placed in a file box for ready reference and the child's own dictionary. Since forgetting recently learned words is very characteristic of dyslexic children, frequent reviews of the old words are essential. If a word is not readily recognized during these reviews, the card is taken out of the file and added to the active file of drill words. Children with severe reading problems often are at the mercy of extraneous clues, pictorial in nature usually, but often they will memorize spots on a card that give the clue to the word. Cards should therefore be rewritten from time to time, possibly with different colored pencils or pens or on different cards. No picture must accompany the words on the cards! Example:

The systematic approach to remediation, not to exceed 15 to 20 minutes per session, must include some record keeping, which should be shared with the child. This method allows for certain reinforcement of learned material and gets the child involved in the entire remedial procedure. A suitable chart for this purpose is reproduced below.

On the following pages in this chapter, some methods of a more specific and inclusive nature are described. Most methods concern themselves with reading, but some are

WEEKLY CHART

Name: .... Week of: ....

Day	Work	Reward
Monday	Words starting with br and bl, like brown and blue. 5 words of each sound blend.	*
Tuesday	Exercise Book, page 56 (left-right exercises). Finished whole page.	**
Wednesday	Practiced th sound, writing th at beginning, middle, and end of words (the/brother/teeth).	*
Thursday	Daddy read story about cowboys. Picked up all words with th sound. Missed 6.	*
Friday	Flash cards, sh sound. Perception exercises, Exercise Book page 57. Work done very well.	***
Saturday	Flash cards, sound sh and ch. Did not recall 10 words from previous day.	*
Sunday	Read all signs in church with Dad and Mom. Spelled and wrote 5 words about church.	**

Total Stars: 11

Note: Keeping a daily log helps in a systematic approach to remedial instructions and keeps track of progress. In addition, it provides for reinforcing (rewarding) the learner as an incentive for improvement. At the end of the day or week, the learner receives his reward in accordance with the tutor's judgment or amount and quality of work performed. Small trinkets and tokens may be used which can be cumulative and exchanged for larger prizes.

also applicable to the remediation of writing, spelling, and arithmetic difficulties. The list of methods is not all-inclusive but contains examples of the more widely known methods in use today. Inclusion of a given method does not necessarily mean endorsement of the method, nor should omissions of other existing methods be construed as disapproval. The methods are described only in an abstract form to familiarize the reader with their basic approach and techniques. Further references on the respective methods are given at the end of each section.

The Orton-Gillingham Method

Samuel T. Orton, a neurologist and often referred to as the father of dyslexia in America, pioneered in the investigation of the nature of developmental language disorders in children and methods of treatment. In 1925 he identified a syndrome of developmental reading disability. Anna Gillingham, a psychologist, was assigned the task of organizing a step-by-step method of remedial instructions for teachers, which has been presented in the Gillingham-Stillman Manual of Remedial Training. The method is based upon visual-auditory-kinesthetic training, called the VAK method for short.

Orton's retraining method, which is also extended to spelling and handwriting, requires the pupil to sound out and trace the visually printed word. Training usually starts with the teaching of basic language units (individual letters and phonemes) and strengthening the visual and auditory patterns by introducing motor elements of speech and writing at the same time. Using step-by-step progressions, the pupil is gradually prepared for longer units, such as more syllables, phrases, and whole sentences.

Orton-Gillingham materials include phonic drill cards for reading and spelling, phonic word cards, graded series of phonetic stories, and other exercises designed to improve reading. In teaching the letters, each phonetic unit is presented on a separate card with consonant letters on white cards and vowel letters on salmon-colored cards. After a list of letters is learned, emphasis is placed on the process of blending as the basis for reading.

Samuel T. Orton, *Reading, Writing, and Speech Problems in Children.* New York: Norton Company, 1937. Reprinted by the Orton Society as Monograph No. 1, rev. 1967.

Materials and publications available from:

The Orton Society, Inc., 8415 Bellona Lane, Suite 115, Towson, MD 21204.

Educators Publishing Service, Inc., 75 Moulton Street, Cambridge, Mass., 02138 (books, tests, and instructional materials).

The Neurological-Impress Method

The Neurological-Impress Method is basically a system of unison reading whereby the student and the teacher read together, aloud, at a fairly rapid rate. The physical arrangement calls for the student to be placed slightly in front of the tutor, both holding the book in their hands. The text is then read in unison, with the voice of the teacher being directed into the ear of the student at close range. The tutor uses the finger of her free hand to locate words and to slide along the line being read. The voice of the tutor is varied as to loudness and softness according to the student's need and proficiency. The approach to the reading is spontaneous, with no special preparations prior to the session. The goal is to read as many pages as possible within a given time limit. No sounds or letters are taught, and no pictorial clues are given or observed. Positive motivation and stimulation are permitted during the reading sessions. The method tries to break down the "phonics-bound" conditions in poor readers, those who have had intensive phonetic training but could not benefit from it. The method is still in an experimental stage, but some research evidence exists. The method claims to avoid erroneous reading habits which may have been imprinted into the child and which cannot be corrected easily once learned. Thus the child has constant positive feedback while reading with the tutor. It appears that this approach is particularly suited for parents and tutors who have no specific background in teaching reading but want to help a poor reader.

R. G. Heckelman, "A Neurological-Impress Method of Remedial-Reading Instructions." *Academic Therapy Quarterly.* Vol. 4, No. 4, 1969, pp. 277–282.

R. G. Heckelman, "The Phonics-Bound Child." *Academic Therapy Quarterly.* Vol. I, No. 1, 1965, pp. 12–13.

K. Lanford, K. Slade, and A. Barnett, "An Examination of Impress Techniques in Remedial Reading." *Academic Therapy.* Vol. IX, No. 5, 1974.

VAKT   (*Visual, Auditory, Kinesthetic, Tactile*)

Dr. Grace M. Fernald, originator of the VAKT method, asserts that difficulty in reading and writing relates directly to defects of sensual perception. Children affected by such defects are often unable to learn in the usual manner and must be taught with reinforcement of other sense modalities such as the visual, auditory, kinesthetic, and tactile. The approach is widely used in Special Education classes in the schools.

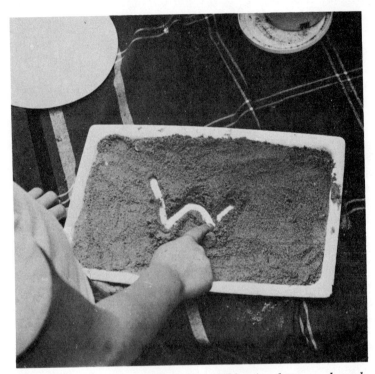

The VAKT Method in action: *The child writes letters and words in a sand tray for tactile-kinesthetic reinforcement of visual or audiovisual clues. Household salt or grits may be substituted for sand. The child "graduates" when he is allowed to write on tabletops or on floor rugs. The idea is that the surface is rough, to be felt easily with the fingers. The Montessori method uses sandpaper for the same purpose.*

Dr. Fernald's objectives are that the child find some way to write words, be motivated to read these words, and then extend his reading to other materials. Typed printing is recommended for these exercises. Each child should be given reading prescriptions that benefit him most. Tracing of words is employed by this method—the child says the letter or word while he is tracing it with his finger. Lexicography (collecting words) is also employed. The words are placed in an alphabetical file for later reidentification. Words are written as whole units and not copied part by part. Children must be taught the meaning of each new word learned. Picture clues are placed on the back of the cards as a reward after the word has been read correctly by the child. Depending on the child's specific areas of deficiency, the VAKT method should be used selectively.

Grace M. Fernald, *Remedial Techniques in Basic School Subjects.* New York: McGraw-Hill Book Company, 1943.

Words-in-Color

The Words-in-Color method was developed by C. Gattegno in England. Because the English alphabet has only 26 characters while the English language has over 200 sounds, Gattegno attempted to phoneticize the alphabet without changing the traditional construct of a single character. By giving each sound a specific color and each letter combination with like sounds the same color, Gattegno has grouped the alphabet and its many combinations phonetically and according to a color coding system. The method employs colored word charts with phonic codes and centers around memorizing phonetic sounds by the color attributed to them. Learning is reinforced with reading booklets, workbooks, word transformation games, word-building books, and a book of stories. While the wall charts are in color, transfer of the various sounds to the workbooks is done in black and white.

C. Gattegno. Words-in-Color (principles of background and teacher's guide). Encyclopedia Britannica Press, 1962.

Materials available from:

Learning Materials, Inc., 100 East Ohio Street, Chicago 11, Ill.

The Montessori Method of Reading

Dr. Maria Montessori was the physician/educator who developed a method for training orphaned and mentally retarded children in the Children's Home in Rome, Italy. Even though Montessori's approach addresses itself to the total development of a child, stressing independence, structure, and perceptual development primarily, the system itself includes a specific method of teaching children how to read. Thus it is not to be considered a single method of remedial instruction.

Montessori felt that writing comes before reading and sought to teach the child, through phonetics, a cursive style alphabet, after which she discovered that spoken words can be analyzed into sounds representing symbols (letters) already learned. The child begins to assemble words phonetically from cardboard letters and then retraces these letters with a pen and paper. Writing and reading exercises are a part of the method. The basic steps in reading acquisition are: (1) mastery of the phonetically learned alphabet; (2) tactile tracing of letters until writing is spontaneous; (3) word recognition from a phonetic sequence of vowels and consonants; (4) interpretation of a sequence of words with meaning; and (5) final active reinforcement. Montessori's approach was translated into many languages and eventually came to America. It requires trained teachers and also calls for specifically designed equipment. Many schools pick out certain aspects of the method and incorporate them into existing approaches to teaching reading.

Maria Montessori, *The Montessori Method*. New York: Schocken Books, 1964.

E. M. Standing, *Maria Montessori: Her Life and Her Work*. New York: New American Library, 1957.

For materials:

A. Daigger and Company, Inc.
Educational Teaching Aid Division
159 West Kinzie Street
Chicago, Ill. 60610

The Ba-Be-Bi Method (Tien's AEIOU&Y Method of Reading)

The rationale underlying the AEIOU&Y method developed by Dr. H. C. Tien, a psychiatrist, is the theory of pattern recognition by identity, which attempts to explain the human brain as a cross-correlation pattern recognition system in the cybernetic sense. Simply speaking, it means that incoming signals have to be recognized by the brain, but to do so we must have the signal of incoming patterns already stored in our brain. To recognize the pattern (letter or word), we must know the pattern.

The method is based on a set of phonetic tables. It uses the conventional alphabet of 26 letters to approximate sounds of English. There are seven basic tables, of which three are used to teach the child to read, but only the First Consonant Table is necessary to get the child started on the road to reading. This table is learned by looking, writing, and saying all combinations at once to produce the basic English syllables. The First Consonant Table is a simple diagram showing all vowels in a row on top of the page (AEIOU&Y), and all single consonants on the left side (*b—c—d*—etc.). Now the child begins to make all possible sound combinations with vowels and consonants, for example, *ba-be-bi-bo-bu-by*; hence the nickname of the method, Ba-Be-Bi. The next table is the Double Consonant Table and has consonant blends in the margin, yielding such combinations as *bla*, *ble*, *bli*, *blo*, *blu*, and *bly*. Worksheets are available for the child to do his exercises, which are very rigid and systematic in nature.

The advantage of the method can be seen in its theoretical foundings and systematic thoroughness—the rigid teaching of the phonetic system in its completeness. The learning of meaning is only secondary in the acquisition of reading. Tien actually states that mothers should be handed his tables the day the baby is born, as an inoculation against reading failure. He also advocates that the pediatrician prescribe a plastic alphabet by the time the child is two years of age.

H. C. Tien, "The AEIOU&Y Method of Reading: Theory and Technique." *Journal of Special Education*, Vol. 1, No. 3, 1967, pp. 223–240.

H. C. Tien, *Reading by Inoculation with the AEIOU&Y Method*. East Lansing, Mich.: Psychodiagnostic Test Company, 1964.

The Initial Teaching Alphabet

The Initial Teaching Alphabet (i.t.a.) was developed by Sir James Pitman in England for use in British schools and is in his words "not a new method of teaching, but a new medium of teaching." In contrast to our 26-letter alphabet, i.t.a. contains 44 symbols—24 of the Roman letters (no q and x), plus 20 new symbols which are mostly typographically linked digraphs. Each of the symbols represents only one sound, and the sound is taught, rather than the letter name. Only lower-case letters are used. A larger version of the lower case is used for capital letters.

a gæm ov baull[1]

British experimentations with the method have tried to demonstrate that i.t.a. not only accelerates progress and raises reading standards, but also raises self-confidence and allows for more independence in work. The child shows marked improvement in creative writing because his thoughts are permitted to flow more naturally in writing. The critical moment comes when the child transfers from i.t.a. to the conventional alphabet, at the end of the third grade. Actually, the i.t.a. system was originally proposed for young children, and it can be used in connection with any method of teaching reading. It is not intended as a universal cure for all reading ills, since it also requires certain preparations and skills from the teacher as well as the use of special materials. It is interesting to note that the originator, Sir James Pitman, did not restrict i.t.a. by copyright. At best, it is a promising innovation which needs further research and development. It is doubtful whether a lay tutor or parent can use the materials without specialized training, but in the hands of a competent teacher it may well be a successful enterprise.

[1] From the book *Early-to-Read*, by Mazurkiewicz and Tanzer, copyright 1963 by Initial Teaching Alphabet Publications, Inc. Reprinted by permission of Pitman Publishing Company.

A. J. Mazurkiewicz and H. J. Tanzer, *Early-to-Read: i/t/a Program*. New York: Initial Teaching Alphabet Publications, Inc., 1963. This is the American source for the dissemination of i.t.a. materials.

J. Downing "Current Misconceptions about i.t.a." *Elementary English*, May 1965

The Sullivan Approach (Programmed Reading Series)

The Programmed Reading Series, developed by Dr. M. W. Sullivan, Cynthia Buchanan and Sullivan Associates, has its major thrust as a linguistic approach, including phonetics and word recognition. The method exists now as a program from the prereading level through the sixth grade. One of the outstanding characteristics of the series is its programmed, step-by-step approach that allows the child to work relatively independently and introduces him systematically into the beginnings of reading. The workbooks are attractive and appeal to children. The approach differs from conventional materials, as it uses discrete words and sentences with humorous illustrations but does not have complete stories in the conventional sense.

C. D. Buchanan and Sullivan Associates, *Programmed Reading*. New York: McGraw-Hill Book Company, 1963.

The selective enumeration and brief description of specific methods of teaching reading given above is intended to give the reader a survey of existing approaches and techniques. Employing these methods for home or classroom use would entail the purchase of some materials which are often not inexpensive, especially if they are used for one or few children. Most methods choose the phonetic approach to teaching reading, either totally or partially. This points out the shortcoming of our English language: If English were 100 percent phonetic, a basically phonetic method would be the most logical approach to teaching reading. But English is not 100 percent phonetic! And the tone-deaf or phonetically insensitive or auditorily handicapped child would be severely penalized if a school used the phonics approach as the sole method of teaching children to read. This is part of the dilemma of the dyslexic child.

The survey of specialized methods, however selective, for teaching the dyslexic child has shown that these methods widely overlap in their approaches. For instance, the use of tracing exercises is *not* unique to one method. Therefore, a choice of methodology can often deteriorate into a "fetish" type or status symbol. "My child attends a Montessori school" can be a very prestigious remark over a cup of tea during the cocktail hour, and the "XYZ" school, which chargse a fee in excess of the average annual salary, can be a mark of distinction to the parents, rather than a school for children with specific learning disabilities.

Teaching methods may also be supplemented with other approaches, as an adjunct to the primary method. The next chapter will discuss some of these treatment procedures and newer methods, to complete the entire spectrum of remedial work in this field.

9 · SECONDARY EMOTIONAL REACTIONS IN DYSLEXIC CONDITIONS

The misery of the dyslexic child actually starts as he enters school. During the early years of childhood he appears as normal and as happy as other children. He may even be promoted to the next higher grade if he has been able to memorize words and sentences in the primer and give them back to the teacher "as if he were reading." Having pictures next to some words or paragraphs in his primer likewise helped him to pretend that he can "read." If he notices a picture of an ax but he says *hatchet*—well, other children in the class also make some mistakes.

As the child begins to experience failure, secondary emotional reactions gradually show up in his behavior. These behaviors are not the beginning of primary emotional disturbances, but are secondary reactions to his budding learning disability. Once remediation is begun on an intensive basis, these reactions usually diminish, but the older the child at the beginning of tutorial efforts, the more chronic these reactions will be, leaving their marks on the general behavior pattern and personality. Under these circumstances it would be quite normal to react in this way because any "handicapped" person would show similar maneuvers to hide his condition, especially in social situations. It is important that parents and educators daily surrounding the child recognize some of these reactions.

The Child's Reactions

The following descriptions of some of these by-products of the dyslexic dilemma are illustrative of how some children show their secondary emotional reactions to a primary learning disability:

1. *Defense and Avoidance Mechanisms.* Defensiveness is evoked in these children when embarrassment has to be avoided among peers or in school situations. This defensive attitude can run the entire gamut from pretending the loss of eyeglasses, misplacing the report card, or showing up late in class when everybody has already had his turn at reading. A boy once told this author that a school bus had run over his lunchbox, which unfortunately, contained his report card. Falsifying one's report card and changing ominous F's to more acceptable C's and D's are also common maneuvers in this category. The defense mechanisms are needed des-

perately to cover up embarrassment and maintain self-respect in the eyes of others. But deep inside, it hurts.

2. *Compensatory Mechanisms.* The mechanisms underlying compensatory maneuvers require a change in behavior. This change is an attempt to substitute for something the poor reader cannot do: namely, read. These compensatory behaviors again run a wide gamut and may be either positive or negative on the surface. Clowning and bragging provoke the attention of peers and may cause the child to be labeled a behavior problem by the teacher, but the behavior is secretly admired by his classmates. Dressing in flashy clothes is another way to compensate. The compensatory mechanism provides the child with some sort of relief, again allowing him to maintain a certain self-respect on the outside while he is suffering inside.

3. *Aggressive Tendencies.* The best defense is attack, as the military knows. Aggression may be expressed overtly in actual fistfights, or covertly by making biting remarks behind the teacher's back. Overt aggression brings immediate attention, while the covert type is sneakier and more self-satisfying. The aggressive tendencies may be interpreted as showing the world that he *can do* something and be superior in some areas, even though they are generally unacceptable socially.

4. *Anxiety and Withdrawal Tendencies.* These secondary emotional reactions are usually found in children who are already anxious and insecure, but the continued failure pattern with academic work intensifies these feelings of anxiety. In reaction to their failures, these children may have nightmares before a reading lesson or the task of standing in front of the entire class to read a story. At other times they may simply not show up for class. School phobias are one

type of reaction, but a phobic reaction is usually an irrational response to an imagined obstacle. In dyslexic children, these obstacles are all too often real and not imagined. The mere appearance of the teacher in class with a reading book under her arm may trigger off these fears and consequent anxiety reactions. Excuses to go to the hall for a drink of water or to go to the rest room are suspiciously frequent and not based on physiological needs.

These secondary emotional reactions can be observed in the human figure drawings made by dyslexic children. The drawings are often characteristic of their behavioral reaction patterns and reflect unconscious feelings. The underlying theme is that of a poor or lowered self-image, sometimes resulting in distorted or grotesque representations of their own self-image. These drawings can be helpful to the professional who attempts a diagnosis of these children based on evaluations and observations. The child with developmental immaturity as the underlying cause of his dyslexia will draw an immature human figure, characteristic of those drawn by much younger children. Organic factors, including minimal cerebral dysfunction (MCD), as a possible cause also may show telltale signs. Another category is a grotesque drawing, sometimes accompanied by obvious or hidden humor. Aggressive/withdrawing tendencies may be observed in drawings where the child has resorted to this kind of reaction to emotional hurts. The following illustrations reveal secondary emotional reactions in children diagnosed as being dyslexic.

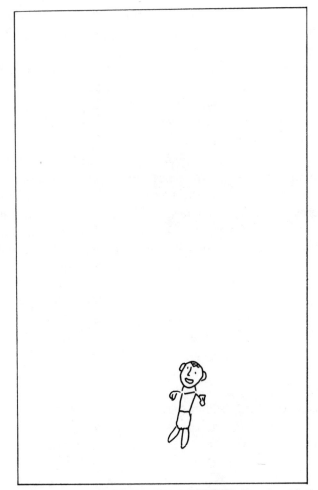

Developmental immaturity *is expressed in this drawing of a nine-year-old boy with dyslexia. He is left-handed, left-eyed, and left-footed, and has a lisp. Reversal errors abound in his reading and spelling. His positioning of the drawing on the sheet of paper reflects shyness and meekness.*

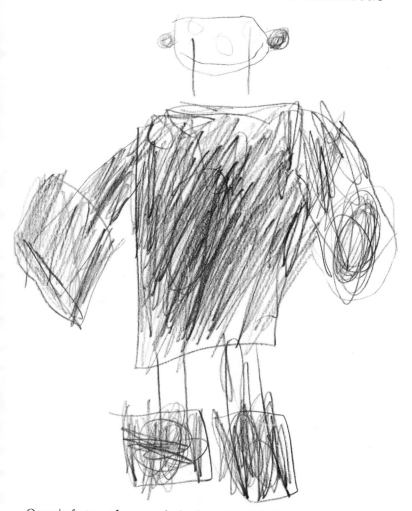

Organic factors *play a marked role in this drawing by an eight-year-old boy who had open-heart surgery with subsequent brain damage. His drawing shows his inner drivenness in heavy line drawing and the blackening in of empty spaces to get rid of his drives and tensions.*

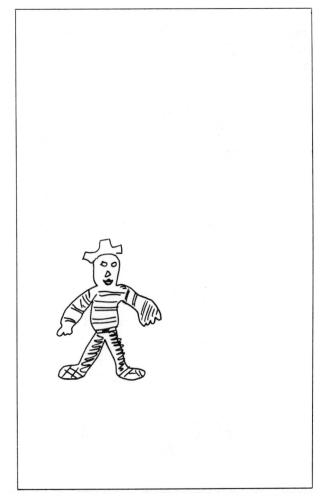

138

Bizarreness *characterizes this drawing by a ten-year-old boy with dyslexia. He wishes to be mummified so that people won't be able to see him and his poor schoolwork. It is almost grotesque.*

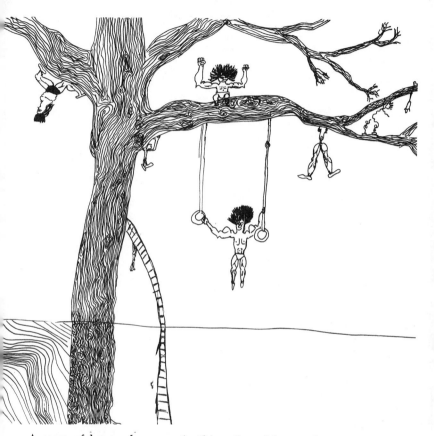

A sense of humor *lures one in this rather elaborate drawing by a twelve-year-old boy with dysgraphia. He cannot write legibly, and his handwriting samples show slanting and difficulties with loops and dots, but these children often compensate with superior drawing ability where creative expression is needed, free from designs to be copied with accuracy (which they cannot do).*

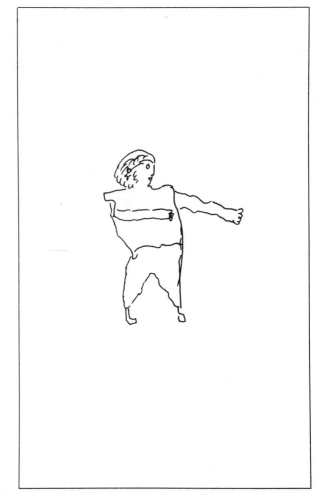

An aggressive stance *marks this drawing by a boy aged fourteen with an IQ of 107 (high average). An eighth-grader reading on the fourth-grade level, he also shows numerous reversals in his oral reading. The aggressive stance seems to symbolize his attitude, as a secondary emotional reaction to his primary learning disability.*

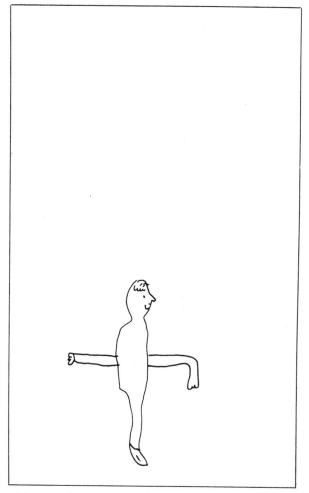

The self-image *of this poor reader, eleven years old and male, in-dicates the spatial disorientation some of the children with LD conditions have. Barely reading on the third-grade level, this youngster also shows numerous reversals (disorientations in space) in his reading. He still confuses* d *and* b, *and reads* bib *for* did, *and* silt *for* slit.

Parental Reactions

Parental or parent surrogates' reactions frequently follow the situations aptly described in terms of transactional analysis (TA) or "games." The idea of playing games—of unconsciously following self-protective patterns of actions or reactions in social situations—was originated by Eric Berne and his associates in California. The TA system allows for simplicity of language used in analyzing behavior. There are three categories of games that parents of dyslexic children often play, with several variations and versions in each of the categories.

1. *Victim Games.* In victim games, the parents feel that they have been "victimized." Someone has given them a dirty deal. They see themselves as martyrs to circumstance rather than to their own failures. The games include "Kick Me!," "Poor Me!," or "Wooden Leg," and they are played as often as applicable. They don't attack those they feel are responsible for their child's dilemma; they simply react as defeatists and act out the game.

2. *Persecutor Games.* These games reinforce the psychological life position of "Not O.K." by reflecting either anger or purity. Constant arguments between the parents might even try to fix the blame on one side, with the resulting games of "I Told You So!," "Yes, But," or "Oh, No, Not This Again!" Mother thinks that Father is to blame because somewhere a distant relative also has a reading problem. In turn, Father blames Mother for overprotecting and coddling the child during the formative years. Every time someone from the school calls, they feel sure people are often after them, out to get them, when they already suffer the miseries associated with a poor learner in the family.

3. *Rescuer Games.* In this category, the parents do not intend to make the confession that they are to blame, that they are "Not O.K." Instead, they try to justify their actions by saying "I'm only trying to help my child" or "Why don't you let me do it for you?" Some teachers, or parents who assist with homework, assume the role of the Great Rescuer, whereby they try to preserve their own integrity, not realizing that in a learning situation *both* parties—the teacher *and* the student, or the parents *and* the child—have to be successful.

School Officials' Reactions

Teachers and principals are human, too, and have their emotional reactions in response to seeing children fail. "Underachiever," "slow learner," "dummy," or "not working up to potential"—all these reactions imply that the student is not doing well because of a suspected low level of intelligence. Another category of reaction is based on the assumption that motivation, or drive, is lacking. "He does not seem to try," "He could do the work if he only tried," or "There are times when I feel he actually can do the work" are commonly encountered remarks. But in children with dyslexic conditions, intellectual competence, at least on low-average levels, is established diagnostically before the label is ever put on them. And as far as motivation goes, some dyslexics try very hard, often doing their homework until past midnight, only to be told the next day in school that their work is unacceptable. Some dyslexics with developmental lags are very slow, and while they can often produce with acceptable accuracy, they lose out because they never finish their work and show up in class the next day with only half of their reading or writing assignments done.

A "Family" Approach to Counseling and Therapy

Remedial intervention other than academic therapy is usually essential in children with dyslexia. They have to be made to feel good about themselves to bring up their low and debasing self-image—the way they feel about themselves. And parents and educators need help, too, because they also have feelings about themselves above and beyond their concern for the child.

Therapeutic treatment of secondary emotional reactions in response to primary learning disabilities is possible but very hard to obtain in some localities. Clinic-type settings with a variety of professional workers on the staff are probably better equipped and better trained than a single professional unless he specializes in these conditions. What is needed is an assessment of *all three parties* involved by getting them together in a counseling situation at least once. This approach has been practiced by the author for many years now and holds high promise of success. The approach is based on the idea of a "multiple image merger hypothesis," in which the three images (child, parents, and educator) are separately assessed and evaluated and brought together (merged) with the aim of obtaining agreement. The process is described elsewhere in more detail.*

In order to get a rough estimate of a child's perception of himself, the How About Me? questionnaire reproduced below may be helpful. A teacher or counselor can ask the questions recorded on the left. While a numerical evaluation is possible, it might be best to inspect the answers only, and get some overall impression of the child's perception of himself. If his answers are mostly in the 4 and 5 categories, we know he needs help. What kind of help is available?

* R. F. Wagner, *Modern Child Management*. Johnstown, Pa.: Mafex Associates, 1975. Softcover edition.

HOW ABOUT ME?

Scale Developed by
R. F. Wagner, Ph.D.

Experimental

Rate yourself on a 5-point scale by placing a checkmark (✓) on top of the line over the appropriate number. Value of numbers: 1 = Very Much; 2 = Much; 3 = Average; 4 = Not Too Much; 5 = Very Little or Low. In case of indecision, the checkmark may also be placed in between two numbers.

1   2   3   4   5

1. How smart are you?

2. How well are you doing in school?

3. How well are you getting along with your classmates?

4. How well are you getting along with adults or grown-ups?

5. How well are you getting along with your parents?

6. What do you think about your health? Do you feel good all of the time?

7. How well do you think you have yourself under control?

8. What about being late getting up or keeping things in order?

9. Are you interested and want to do things in school?

10. Do you have lots of energy? Are you a go-getter? And always on the go?

Remediation and Therapy

Remediation efforts and treatment of secondary emotional reactions to primary learning disabilities are possible but hard to obtain in a given locality. Here are some of the possibilities, depending on the child's symptomatology, availability of treatment, and financial ability of the parents:

Tutorial Relationship. In special classroom situations or in 1:1 pupil/teacher relationships, the low ratio is often given credit for improvements. However, it appears that the close relationship is very conducive to the incidental treatment of secondary emotional reactions and requires teacher qualifications in both the academic and counseling areas.

Supportive Counseling. Supportive counseling should be a concomitant of specialized tutoring and academic remediation. It might be as important for the parents as it is for the child, and can be carried out by the school counselor or school psychologist.

Psychotherapy. In severe cases of emotional reactions, professional psychotherapy is indicated, usually provided by psychiatrists and well-trained psychologists.

Medication. Medication is prescribed by qualifed physicians only, often as an adjunct to ongoing academic remediation, counseling, or psychotherapy. At this stage, drug therapy still lacks the specificity needed to remedy the problem of learning or reading per se. At best a child may be made amenable to the ongoing remediation or treatment. The hyperactive child may calm down, or the anxious might become less anxious, in order to benefit from specialized tutoring. The most frequently prescribed drug seems to be Ritalin, indicated, among several other conditions, for functional behavior problems in children (hyperactivity, stuttering, and so on).

Behavior Modification. In recent years, special conditioning procedures have been used successfully with all types of behavior, including learning disabilities. The advantage of the method lies in its precision and specificity. The behavior of whole classrooms may be modified, or the method can be applied to an individual child by rewarding certain bits or small units of behavior which are already in the child's repertoire but whose frequency should be increased, for example, attention span or time attending to a given task.

Curriculum Modification. Whether or not a dyslexic child should remain in his classroom or be isolated into special group or class situations is still controversial. One of the advantages of remaining in the regular class is that the child can stay with his age group, possibly lessening the emotional reactions he has to learning. On the other hand, he may become more sensitive to class reactions and will resort to some of the symptoms described earlier. Both strategies have merit.

New and Controversial Treatments

Fortunately, research is actively pursued in the area of learning disabilities. These studies are often carried by one specialty, or they may involve a multidisciplinary approach, where, for example, medicine combines with psychology to delve into the hidden mysteries of LD conditions. Since these are research studies, they are often limited in scope and methodological approach and therefore the results cannot be generalized immediately. In many cases, so-called replication studies have to be carried out in order to verify initial findings. In other instances, double-blind studies are made to hide the identity of the researcher as well as the treatment so that objective data can be obtained. Among treatments and therapies currently in vogue, but not yet fully proved, are the following.

Food additives are often suspected of being the major cause of hyperactivity—or hyperkinesis, as the medical profession calls the condition. Foods containing additives, dyes, or salicylates are to be excluded from the diet of the learning-disabled child, according to this theory. One of the investigators of this theoretical view is Dr. Benjamin Feingold. This diet theory is currently being researched extensively.

Brain allergies are based on the hypothesis that the brain may be hypersensitive to certain foods and chemicals. Some children suffer from fatigue, irritability, stomachaches, and other symptoms. Apparently, some of these cases respond to antihistamine treatment or other forms of chemotherapy for allergies. Obviously, some of these symptoms may contribute to poor school performance, and if these symptoms are relieved, improved academic work may result.

Hypoglycemia is also suspected as a cause of LD conditions. The intake of sweets, especially in the morning during breakfast, leads to an abrupt rise in the blood sugar level. This, in turn, stimulates the pancreas to secrete insulin, which brings the blood sugar level down again. Low blood sugar conditions are said to interfere with certain brain functions and are symptomatically related to poor school performance. Adherents to this theory would advise parents to use sugar moderately through strict dietary control.

Megavitamins or *megavitamin therapies* use massive doses of vitamins that supposedly provide each cell in the body, including the brain, with the optimum environment of chemicals. Megavitamin therapy is used in a variety of illnesses and conditions, and is also employed under medical supervision in the treatment of learning disabilities and psychoses in children. No conclusive evidence exists that the treatment is totally effective. Another mode of treatment is with *trace minerals*, in which an analysis of the hair reveals certain mineral imbalances.

In addition to the above novel approaches, some provoking great controversies in this country among professionals, we find an array of *neurophysiologic-retraining* methods prevalent among treatments being tried out by researchers. *Patterning*, for example, is based on a theory that failure to pass through certain sequences of developmental stages reflects poor neurological organization. The child is then "patterned," or retrained, by going through various movements, such as crawling. Another treatment is known as *sensory integrative therapy*, and there are also various approaches to *optometric training*.

While the reader has been offered a variety of new and sometimes controversial methods and treatments, their enumeration does not represent endorsement here. As with all new ideas and new treatment modes, caution is advisable. Only a trusted professional should make the referral.

The last word has not yet been spoken regarding the identification, remediation, and prevention of specific reading disabilities. Teachers are being trained in specialized methods, research is going on in this field with more intensified effort than before, and federal funds are gradually pumped into projects, schools, and research centers. But new children with dyslexia are discovered every day, and they need help at once. Until a panacea is found, reading problems are here to stay.

10 · DYSLEXIA AND
THE ADOLESCENT

When the noted psychoanalyst Eric Erikson states that normal adolescents undergo an *identity crisis*, how much more must it affect the dyslexic, who is under constant stress. A young man aged thirty told the author about the trials and tribulations he had to undergo as a dyslexic, reading on the second-grade level. "It was hell in school," he stated, "with a constant vigilant attitude so that people wouldn't find out that I couldn't read." Term papers and book reports were copied from a buddy on the way to school. It was a "hide-and-seek" game that put him under constant stress. After leaving school—he dropped out in the ninth grade after repeating a grade three times—he hopped from one job to another, always afraid someone might discover his dyslexia and embarrass him. "One day I got a job, or I thought I got it, in a fast-food service place, but they handed me an application form to fill out, so I ran home quickly and had my twelve-year-old daughter fill it out for me. Then I ran back to the place and handed it to the manager. I was supposed to be the cook, and even though I knew damn well how to cook hamburgers, the man took me in the back and showed me a slide show on how to prepare hamburgers. But then he handed me a quiz, a piece of paper with questions written on it, and I was to fill it out and answer the test questions. I sat there for a while, like a dummy, and then I asked to be excused. I told him I had to go to the rest room. But I walked right by the rest room, out on the street where I had my car parked, and I drove off without ever returning there."

While a few people and public agencies are slowly becoming aware of the problem that presents itself when a person cannot read properly, the dilemma still exists. A recent newspaper article related the story of a young Navy recruit who entered the service after completing high school and one year of junior college. But he was reading at the second-grade level. He was assigned to an intensive five-week course in reading conducted by a petty officer, and reportedly improved by nearly three grades after completing the course. That improvement was sufficient to open up a few opportunities, starting with admission to basic training. The spokesman for the Navy stated that they can do a better job at teaching reading than public schools because they have better discipline, better instructors in front of the kids all the time, and they supervise their homework. It does not speak too well for our public schools. Why don't they have better discipline and better instructors, and why don't they supervise homework?

In another newspaper report recently, a would-be robber with sloppy handwriting was arrested because the bank teller said she couldn't decipher the stick-up note and told him to write another one that was readable. While he did, she pushed the silent alarm. Dysgraphia just does not pay off!

Favorable and Unfavorable Conditions for Teaching the Dyslexic

The picture of making another attempt to teach the growing child who has become a teenager is not completely unfavorable. For instance, in older children hyperactivity begins to slow down and level off. They are no longer home- and office-wreckers. They are able to sit down and look at a book. If they have undergone such unfortunate experiences as those described above, they are ready to have another crack at it. In other words, motivation is no longer a problem, provided they can find someone, somewhere, who is able and willing to teach them. But to find this someone is difficult, and almost impossible in some situations or smaller communities.

Another favorable feature is that the adolescent and young adult have matured. Parents have been reminded that "Johnny will outgrow it," but maturation was slow and took years, as one would expect it to do. But while there are many significant changes in the budding adult, such as physical, hormonal, and psychological ones, certain growth phenomena disappear because maturation has set in. Silly defense mechanisms have finally been given up, but sometimes they have only changed to different ones, often in the disguise of games. A young man told the author recently that he used to run away in school when someone confronted him with a reading task. Now he tries to invent maneuvers to stay on the scene and ward off embarrassment through trickery. If someone hands him a piece of paper with a joke on it, he will pass it to someone else in the crowd and say, "Here, read it first!" and then wait for that person's reaction. If he laughs, so does our poor reader. If he says nothing, our poor reader also copies that reaction. Pitiful? Yes!

One of the unfavorable conditions is that the family by now has given up on the adolescent dyslexic. They have tried everything, have consulted "experts" and spent money by the buckets—to no avail. Even if the dyslexic has received some help in the past and has improved slightly, he is again confronted with a dilemma because his peers have progressed according to normal levels while he has remained behind, falling back because no one has bothered to reinforce what was so hard for him to acquire in the first place. Unless a dyslexic condition is continuously reinforced by suitable exercises, what has been gained is quickly lost. A young man entering college after receiving some training for his dyslexia will once again face failures because he has not kept up with his skills and is far behind the others.

By now, the self-image of our adolescent dyslexic is at a bottom level. He has no confidence in himself when it comes to reading, or spelling, or what not, because he has incorporated this failure pattern into his life-style. If a dyslexic condition remains untreated, the secondary emotional reactions come to the fore more markedly and often are part of the entire personality pattern of the individual.

And there is more that is unfavorable. Due to the continued learning disability, the young person has been unable to take advantage of the environment, which normally provides him with the input of material that a person has to stash away in his memory storage on a long-term basis. In childhood, we learn basic information, facts and figures, which we need on a maintenance basis and will have to recall later. Complicated math problems cannot be solved unless one also knows the basic concepts. Concepts cannot be understood on a verbal level unless one is familiar with basic data and information. The adolescent dyslexic lacks this storage and thus has few facts in his memory bank to draw on. As a result, test scores go down, including those on the intelligent test (IQ). If someone tries to feed him this needed information orally, perhaps via tape recordings, he may be better off. At least he can retrieve what was put into his memory by ear. But the information that could have been obtained through the eyes, that is, by reading, is not readily available and presents a real deficiency—a vacuum, a void, a gaping abyss.

Career Choices and Vocational Guidance

Vocational guidance can become a key factor in the life of someone who does not possess adequate reading skills. What if the reading disability remains undetected, or remedial efforts were not fully rehabilitative, and the young adolescent does not read on minimally acceptable levels? Granted, there are jobs in which reading is not a specific requirement, but the dyslexic has a right to dream and choose according to his wishes and desires. Choosing a career means narrowing down a wide array of possibilities to one job after carefully weighing preference against existing skills and talents. If reading is not one of those skills, the dyslexic's freedom of choice becomes miserably restricted and confined.

Guidance counselors in our schools are poorly prepared to help dyslexics find suitable careers. The reason for this is that they have little specific knowledge of what a learning disability is and what it entails, and they are even less adequately prepared to deal with vocational planning. Yet there are colleges and schools throughout the country that accept applications from handicapped students, including those with learning disabilities. Local chapters of the Association for Children with Learning Disabilities (see the Appendix for its address) often can be very helpful in supplying the necessary information.

Another source that has proved helpful is a program called Vocational Rehabilitation, with state and local offices. Some of the local units are attached to public-school systems and may actually be housed in those systems. The telephone directory can also provide the necessary information. Usually, adolescents become eligible at the age of fifteen, but policies may vary in different localities. In some instances, preventive intervention can be started before the specified age of eligibility. Some agencies provide for diagnostic work-ups only, while others have remedial facilities. In most instances, mental health centers are less well adequately equipped to deal with the problem of dyslexia.

Need for Counseling

If the dyslexic goes through life untreated, secondary emotional reactions will at times become primary; thus, on the behavioral surface the person resembles those peers who display primary symptoms of emotional reactions and even disturbances. The author recalls a thirty-year-old man who ended up in a psychiatrist's office because his deep depressions prevented him from functioning normally. He had been turned down time and again for promotions on his job because of his poor reading, and his little daughter, aged six, had begun to read and was innocently trying to hop on her father's lap to listen to him read her a story from a book. Unable and disenchanted, he withdrew farther and farther from family life. The final breakdown came when someone in church asked him to read a passage from the Bible. Tears came to his eyes as he walked out the back door, and he never stopped walking until he reached the emergency room of the local hospital.

While the foregoing example may be an extreme one, professionals working in the area of learning disabilities could add many more such instances. Lucky is the young man or woman whose father has a business of his own and is able to hire his offspring in some manner. There are times when the dyslexic can enter a vocational career successfully —always avoiding reading, of course—but the dilemma may not start until he decides to marry. The embarrassments intensify as his future spouse begins to wonder about him. Why does he never look at a newspaper? Why is his knowledge of literature so poor? Why does he avoid looking up information in the dictionary? The day of confession approaches and could spell disaster if his fiancée does not understand the situation. And even if she does, what can she do to help him?

The need for counseling is great in all these instances, but specialized help is often unavailable. The key words are *supportive counseling* rather than intensive therapy. The dyslexic needs support, understanding, and acceptance because he is *not* crazy! He is *not* dumb! And he is *not* lazy! He wants to learn, but he can't.

Lack of Facilities

One could not make the statement that there are no facilities in the United States to come to the aid of the dyslexic person, whether child, adolescent, or adult. However, such help does not exist evenly spread out over the entire life of a dyslexic person. Before school, approximately until age four or five, early detection and prevention is hard to come by. Some school systems have effective screening programs, but by no means all. During the kindergarten or first-grade years, facilities may exist, but someone has to notice the symptoms of dyslexia and refer the child to the appropriate source. In elementary schools, facilities are often available and concentrated, with a variety of help in existence, such as a resource room, special reading teachers, and so on.

The adequacy or availability of such services for the dyslexic child begins to thin out, if not to disappear, in junior and senior high school. Most educators would admit that they have help in the elementary grades, but in the higher grades such help is hard to find. There are private schools that specialize in learning disabilities, but their tuition is so forbiddingly high that their facilities are reserved for a few people of means. Some school systems provide tuition grants, with partial or total reimbursement. But in some instances the school system does not agree with the diagnosis and their decisions have to be appealed at the review board or state department level.

The time when the need is the greatest and facilities are almost nonexistent is in adolescence and young adulthood. Only a few—a very few—major cities may have such adult learning centers. Smaller cities and rural areas do not have them. Unless federal or state authorities become aware of these crying needs and provide financing, self-help is about all that is available. There are isolated places where civic organizations have become aware of this and tried to arrange for some self-help.

Appropriateness of Reading Materials

It is not unusual to find an adolescent reading on the third-grade level. If he is diagnosed as a dyslexic, he probably has average or better intelligence but reads much below expectancy. If reading instructions were again begun at such an age and on this level, would one once again have to resort to "Dick and Jane" books or similarly elementary reading materials? It may well be that our dyslexic adolescent is once again turned off by such childish texts. This situation often exists when the teacher is unable to locate suitable textbook material for the older dyslexic. One way of overcoming this situation is to write one's own text on a typewriter, but not every teacher is resourceful and creative enough, not to speak of the extra hours she has to put into such efforts. Only fairly recently have publishers become aware of this need and published textbooks or reading material with low-grade-level and high-motivational content.[1]

A similar situation exists with regard to tests. Test items usually require a knowledge of reading to answer the questions. No wonder, then, that dyslexics come up with poorer scores than their reading counterparts. A dyslexic should not be required to take tests designed for readers. In

[1] For a list of such publishers, see: R. F. Wagner, *Helping the Wordbind. Effective Intervention Techniques for Overcoming Reading Problems in Older Students*, Appendix. West Nyack, N.Y.: The Center for Applied Research in Education, Inc., 1976.

some instances, allowances are made for these deficiencies, but it is not the prevailing attitude in the United States. In some European countries, such as Germany, a dyslexic child is given a small certificate, similar to a credit card, which he presents to the teacher before a test is given. The card certifies him as a legitimate dyslexic and exempts him from the test. Instead, the test is usually given *orally*. The final scores often surprise the educator. A dyslexic can show his true intelligence when the reading barrier is removed.

What Will the Future Bring?

Follow-up research studies are relatively rare because of the time span they entail. So-called longitudinal studies not only require time and someone to live long enough to do them personally or leave them as a legacy to others to continue, but they also entail locating people who may have spread out all over the country and the globe after they leave school. This school leaving might have been a dropping out rather than an honorable graduation with a certificate or diploma to prove it.

One of the more comforting thoughts expressed in this book is the fact that a number of men and women who have had reading problems in their school years have nevertheless proved that they can succeed, whatever the odds against them. Among such people we find Thomas A. Edison, the inventor; Auguste Rodin, the sculptor; Woodrow Wilson, the president; and Hans Christian Andersen, the storyteller. Andersen spelled *Temps* for *Thames* and *brackfest* for *breakfast*. Former Vice-President Nelson Rockefeller was a dyslexic. Dyslexics can be found among physicians, lawyers, insurance salesmen—and butchers, bakers, and candlestick makers.

One of the frequently cited follow-up studies is that by Margaret B. Rawson, who published her study in a book entitled *Developmental Language Disability, Adult Accomplishments of Dyslexic Boys* (The Johns Hopkins University Press, 1968). Rawson's longitudinal investigation of fifty-six boys, some dyslexic and some nondyslexic, provides an encouraging answer to the question of what happens to poor readers after they leave school. It also contradicts the notion that poor readers are incapable of performing well in areas requiring language ability. For a period of approximately thirty years, Rawson followed the education and career development of boys from a private school that was one of the first with a program for the detection of reading disabilities. Perhaps a grain of salt should be used in drawing ultimate conclusions from the results of the study because the sample Rawson used cannot be considered representative or typical of a public-school setting or an "average" American school system.

Under the circumstances Rawson encountered, her study was an objective one. There were twenty boys in the sample who were considered dyslexic, and these were compared with the remaining thirty-six boys in the sample. After examining the sociological and psychometric characteristics of her groups, Rawson ranked them on a composite scale of various characteristics demonstrating language disability. Against this background of accumulated data, she presented the study of the adult accomplishments of each of the fifty-six boys in the sample. And what did she find out?

Dyslexic boys, that is, poor readers with average and above-average intelligence, are not necessarily poor occupational and academic risks. The results of the investigation show that dyslexics are capable of average and even superior achievement in later years. Because verbal skills are so important to educational and vocational success in our modern world, the study should be of great interest to everyone working with learning-disabled youngsters.

In another, even more recent study, Frauenheim[2] reports a study of forty males who were diagnosed as dyslexic in childhood. Reading, spelling, and arithmetic were again tested, with the following results: Severe residual learning problems are present despite the fact that much special attention was provided during the school-age years. The author also observed that the current learning difficulties in the sample of forty men tested were essentially identical to those evidenced at the time of the diagnosis. While this seems to imply the adage that "Once a dyslexic, always a dyslexic," it does not allow for sweeping conclusions at this time, since the sample used in the study represented a very low level of the scale. Lighter cases might fare much better, and a more mature life-style could possibly lessen the problems encountered in the world of work by dyslexic males.

[2] Frauenheim, J. G. Academic Achievement Characteristics of Adult Males Who Were Diagnosed as Dyslexic in Childhood. *Journal of Learning Disabilities*, Vol. 11, No. 8. Oct. 1978, pp. 476–483.

11 · SPECIFIC LEARNING DISABILITIES: AN UMBRELLA CONCEPT

The term *specific learning disabilities* (SLD) is a relative newcomer on the scene of learning problems and does not specify the particular area in which a child may experience problems. Early attention in life is focused on reading problems simply because reading is an all-important ingredient in the learning process. It is difficult for a person to obtain a job later in life unless he can read fluently. Filling out an employment application will reveal other shortcomings because the forms usually ask questions that have to be read first before one can answer them appropriately or correctly. Writing down the answers will also stamp the person with an SLD label because it will bring his faulty spelling to light. And one's handwriting has to be legible unless one is a physician, in which case only the pharmacist has the deciphering problem. Errors in arithmetic, comprehension, and speech are also possible and come under the umbrella concept, but they may not be so readily recognized by the observer. However, the same underlying causes may creep up in the different areas. For example, a child may reverse *on* and *no*, but he may also read *41* as *14*. In spelling, *fashion* and *fashoin* (sic) may look alike to the SLD child.

Another interesting characteristic in SLD conditions is that they may occur in isolation (e.g., reading only), or in combinations. The most commonly observed combination is reading and spelling below expectancy, with arithmetic and thinking relatively high. Poor handwriting may occur in isolation, but it may also be coupled with poor spelling (and in some cases *not* reading!). When a maturational lag is the causative factor for the condition, we often observe its effect in many, if not all, areas of development. A child may have articulatory problems, but may also have a very clumsy grip on the pencil and be below expectancy in reading. In addition, he may not be fully toilet-trained or he may play with much younger children.

The degree of deficit likewise plays a role in judging SLD conditions. A person may not only have deficiencies in particular areas, but they may occur in relative degrees. A student in the sixth grade may read on the fifth-grade level, indicating a milder form of dyslexia, while his comprehension is at the third-grade level, a more serious condition.

Reading (Dyslexia). The preceding chapters have emphasized reading problems because the book is written on this subject and because most parents and educators are interested in this particular area of academic achievement. It is impossible for a student to function adequately in the classroom unless he can read on average levels. If he cannot

SPECIFIC LEARNING DISABILITIES

An Umbrella Concept

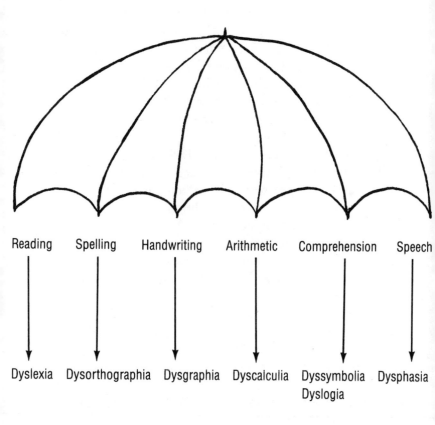

do this, attention will be drawn to his poor performance at once, whether he is singled out for remedial classes or called a "dummy" by his peers.

Even within the narrower category of reading, we have seen that there can be many different things that are deficient. If a child has difficulty with auditory discrimination, that is, he cannot distinguish *pit* and *pet* when he hears the words pronounced by someone, he has difficulties in the auditory perceptual realm and may be diagnosed as having *Auditory Dyslexia*. On the other hand, when visual perceptual problems exist, such as rotation or reversal of single letters or whole words, *Visual Dyslexia* is the problem. The more specifically one can isolate the problem area or areas within a category, the more specifically can the remediation procedures be spelled out. It is also quite possible that a given student has a *mixed* problem, meaning that both phonetic sensitivity (an auditory perception problem) and visual perception are the cause.

But the variety of causative sources does not end here. A child may have trouble with sequencing letters properly within a word (w-o-r-d), or words within an entire sentence (The cat ran fast).

Spelling (Dysorthographia). Poor spelling must be distinguished from poor handwriting. Many half-trained "specialists" do not address themselves to this distinction and treat the condition with one and the same remedial technique. However, a disinction must be made because there are children who have good handwriting but have trouble spelling. On the other hand, there are those children with poor handwriting who spell on acceptable levels. We shall take up poor spelling first.

As in dyslexia, poor spelling may have several possible

causes. A child may be able to spell correctly when the words are dictated to him and he is required to give back the spelling *orally*, without writing the words down. He may do this correctly but make mistakes when asked to write the words down on paper. Apparently, in such situations the child has no auditory difficulties and hears things as said, but begins to confuse the letter sequence and letter symbols when visual perceptions enter the process. A reverse condition is possible but rarely observed in the practical situation. In other instances, sometimes in cases with organic causes, the child focuses on segments of the word structure, such as prefix-stem-suffix, because the field of vision is narrowed. If he has to copy the word from a sample, he introduces unnecessary mistakes. Improper sequencing with resulting transformation errors (for example, *tilt* for *title*) can also be at fault at times. This mixed-up spelling order was observed by Dr. Samuel Orton, an American neurologist, who called the condition *strephosymbolia* (from the Greek, meaning "scrambled symbols"). Reversal errors, such as spelling *musuem* (sic) instead of *museum*, are commonly found among poor spellers.

Handwriting (Dysgraphia). While handwriting styles can be individually different but still within an acceptable range, poor handwriting can be considered an SLD condition. Sometimes people with neurological problems show poor handwriting as a graphic expression of unsteadiness. In European countries the pseudoscience of graphology is practiced for an analysis of character and personality. Most often, poor handwriting is associated with slow or deficient sensorimotor development in children. They have difficulty with tracing and staying within lines when they are young, and later on in school they reveal poor handwriting habits.

The handwriting samples reproduced on pages 168–169 show some of the particular difficulties. Slanting is a major problem. Often the writing is very uneven and may at times lean to the left, at other times to the right, all in the same word or sentence. Looping is another area. Here the child has difficulty making loops, as in cursive *a* or *o*. When letters have to be combined in cursive handwriting (not in printing), loops are of different lengths and frequently run into each other, making reading the sample most difficult for others—and for themselves, for that matter, when they are asked to read their own writing. One of the basic errors is being inconsistent, mixing printing with cursive, or forgetting to cross the *t* or put the dot over the *i*.

In dysgraphic conditions, a multisensory approach to remediation is essential. The child must first *feel* the shape of the letters or words through tactile-sensory modalities. Tracing exercises are also very helpful. However, the parent or educator must exercise patience in the remedial process since dysgraphic conditions require more time for remediation than does reading or even spelling. The inconsistency sometimes pops up in uneven writing, meaning that one day these children write fairly well, while on other days they produce poor writing. The idea of medication, with the help of a physician, as an adjunct therapy is often advisable. A further inconsistency is in mixing up large and small letters. Sentences are often begun in small letters, while a few lines below, the same words are capitalized. Needless to mention, punctuation is another hazard for these children, with colons, semicolons, commas, and periods freely interchanged on a random basis.

Examples of how some dyslexic children write the sentence "Did the man walk on ice?"

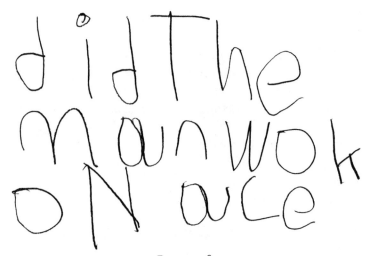

Boy, age 8.

Boy, age 11.

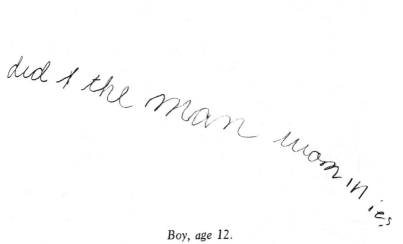

Boy, age 12.

Boy, age 9.

Arithmetic (Dyscalculia). It might not be surprising to see the same errors made in reading, spelling, and handwriting show up in arithmetic. For instance, the reversal phenomenon can be present when a child reads *was* for *saw* but also reads or writes 28 for 82. However, two types of errors are important here and must be viewed separately: visual perception and comprehension, which in this case is called arithmetic reasoning. Modern mathematics has given these children an added burden since they have to *read* lengthy problems before they can proceed to solve them. In addition, modern mathematics requires more thinking than simple numerical manipulations. The problem $3 + 4 = 7$ is different from $3 + n = 7$ because the unknown number n requires a comprehension process that does not exist in the first example.

In addition to the visual-perceptual aspects involved in arithmetic processes, the child's reasoning plays an important role. Conceptual trouble often begins when fractions are introduced. The child may have no idea of what "an eighth" means, and how various fractions can be combined. The positions of numerator and denominator, furthermore, represent orientations in space, another area where the SLD child may have a problem. He may not perceive the difference between $1/4$ and $4/1$. Trouble with comprehension, known as arithmetic reasoning, really starts when the problems are stated *verbally*. How can the child even attempt to find a solution when he has not understood the meaning of the question? The concepts of "carrying" and adding or subtracting from right to left are also problematic to him. In reading, the sequence is from left to right, while in adding and subtracting, the direction goes from right to left. If this is not confusing to the dyscalculic youngster, what is?

Comprehension (Dyssymbolia). In the hierarchy of learning, the basic rung on the ladder is sensorimotor function, followed by perception, imagery, and symbolization, climaxed by concept formation and inferential thinking. Errors in symbolization are therefore of a higher order in the cognitive realm. Symbolization means finding a symbol for an object or situation that has been perceived; an image (auditory or visual) has been established in the mysterious intricacies of the brain, but now we have to narrow the image down to a symbol. The imagined picture of four legs and a flat surface on top is represented by the word *table*. No doubt this symbol will facilitate memorization and recall when we are required sometime later to say the word again. Symbolization improves the efficiency of thinking by finding abbreviations, similar to shorthand, that label situations. Commonly, this is accomplished with words, but there are mathematical concepts that require nonalphabetical symbols, such as "larger than" and "smaller than" ($<$ and $>$).

Where the difficulty for the SLD child comes in is not in the deciphering of the text, as in reading, but in the drawing of inferences and the making of abstractions. "A stitch in time saves nine" gives us distinct words with specific underlying meanings attached to the words, but it requires a cognitive process—abstraction and comprehension—to arrive at the higher meaning, namely *prevention*. "An apple a day keeps the doctor away" has little to do with apples or doctors, for we could substitute bananas or plums, and in the case of a dog we could substitute a veterinarian. Again, the same higher-level concept has to be inferred, namely, "prevention."

By diagnostic assessment, the SLD child possesses at least low-average intelligence, with an IQ around 85 or above, depending on the test given and the classificatory terminology used. Thus, one can expect the child to abstract on a level commensurate with his intelligence. However, in instances of dyssymbolia, it is precisely this aspect of intellectual functioning—comprehension—that is deficient. Not all deficits are at the apex of thinking, such as drawing inferences. Some children show them in as simple an area as knowing opposites; for example, good-bad or smart-stupid. In other cases, the child looks at a butterfly, for example, but cannot tell what it stands for, what it symbolizes (possible answers: freedom, nature, movement, beauty).

In comprehension problems, one finer distinction has to be made. If the child does not have the ability to abstract or think on levels of a higher order, the condition is called *dyssymbolia*. However, in some instances the child *does* have this ability but cannot express it. This is called *dyslogia* (from the Greek *logos*, meaning "word"). A condition in which the child is having difficulty finding a word he wishes to express or understand will be discussed next. Comprehension is a brain action where information is processed, while the next section deals with the inability to recall (express) or understand (receive) words.

Speech (Dysphasia). When a person has difficulty in finding a word or expressing it, whether in speech or the written word, we have a dysphasic condition. The child may try to avoid saying the word by substituting nonfluencies ("ah") or referring to an object as a "doolully" or a "what-you-call-it." In response to the question "What do you do if a child much smaller than you hits you?" he might reply "Annoy him!" when he actually wanted to say "Ignore him!" In another instance, a child might be totally unable to give a reply but will give the correct answer when asked to write it on a sheet of paper. That such incorrect answers affect the score on an intelligence test is obvious. A child may be labeled retarded on the basis of a score thus lowered, when in actuality he could have given the correct answer if he had been asked to write it down.

In conditions in which the sensory input is affected, that is, in which the child does not understand certain words or phrases, the danger of not producing the correct results are even more pronounced. Only a sensitive and well-trained professional will be able to detect such deficiencies and address himself to the problem by making sure that the child understands the question fully. If no other ways and means of adequate communication can be found, a nonverbal test might be used to assess intelligence more adequately. Dysphasic conditions can often be treated by speech therapists and speech pathologists, whose professional training usually includes the treatment of dysphasic and aphasic conditions.

There are more conditions, and often hard-to-detect ones, that fit under our umbrella concept of learning disabilities, but the list is already long enough. For example, a child may have trouble with memory storage (retention) or memory recall (retrieving and/or saying words). Either condition can affect short-term and/or long-term memory. Some children forget words overnight, while others retain them for a few days or weeks, but then forget them completely. Frequent reinforcement would be indicated in such conditions. Poor memorization may be caused by several factors and can affect several modalities. We distinguish between auditory and visual memory, both highly essential ingredients in the reading process. But there are other sensory avenues that can be at fault, such as tactile (touching) and kinesthetic (feeling and orientation in space).

The more specifically the deficiencies or dysfunctions can be diagnostically pinpointed, the more precisely the learning disability can be remediated.

12 · AN OUNCE OF PREVENTION . . . AND THE ACADEMIC SURVIVAL PROGRAM

If a child suffers from a reading deficiency, he is able to view the world only through a half-opened door. Much of the information presented to us through reading is unavailable to him. It is true that not all our information is acquired through reading, but the fact remains that a large proportion is. Another important fact enters the dilemma of the dyslexic here: once the reading deficiency is detected and help secured, the child is bombarded with an overdose of reading instructions. He spends a disproportionate amount of time on remedial reading in order to catch up with his peers, while at the same time he is not receiving the general information taught in a regular curriculum. This becomes a vicious circle, as we shall see instantly.

We have come to realize—after decades of fruitless see-saw argumentation—that tests of intelligence are not solely based on inborn abilities but are also dependent on acquired knowledge gathered after birth. And some intelligence tests contain precisely such questions, which the child can answer only if he has been exposed to an opportunity to learn the facts, such as listening, reading, incidental remarks, records or TV or even advertising. Some children are able to compensate for the blocked reading pathways by listening more carefully than normal children. We know of a physician with a reading deficiency who, as a young medical student, would religiously record the professors' lectures on a tape recorder, or ask some of his fellow students to read the textbooks to him for a modest fee. But not all students are able to compensate successfully for their reading problems. Many are not reached by stimulation that stems solely from reading materials, thus losing out on its valuable contents and information—and tragically so.

The obvious inference here is that if a child was given an intelligence test during his early years, say, at the age of six, seven, or eight, and then retested after a few years, the results of the second test are often lower, due to the lack of exposure to information that other children get through reading. He "loses" IQ points simply because he may not be able to answer such questions as, "Who was Plato?" or, "How far is it from New York to Mexico City?" He cannot answer these "intelligence" questions because he was never exposed to the reading material which would have fed him the needed information. The child was penalized for a lack of opportunity, much as the so-called culturally deprived children have a lack of exposure for which they must pay the price in school. Many may not accept the inference of intelligence from an IQ score; they may claim that it is not a logical step; but this is how our children are judged in school, in many instances. To be on the Honor Roll, to enter a certain fraternity or sorority, to receive scholarships, to impress a teacher, to compete in scholastic competitions —these require a fairly high IQ score. The consequences of such thoughts are detrimental to many poor readers, if not disastrous:

YOUR CHILD might have lowered IQ scores as he progresses through the school grades or grows older, while his reading disability is either undetected or untreated.

YOUR CHILD might be held back a grade or placed in a class for "slow learners" if his scores on standard intelligence tests have become lower over the years.

YOUR CHILD will need more time, much more time, to acquire the knowledge other children already possess, in order to catch up with the others. With luck and hard work he will have caught up in two, three, four years—when the other children have had a head start for further advancing their knowledge.

YOUR CHILD will have to be exposed to sources other than reading material in order to stay abreast of the average reader. Many educators are not aware of this lack of opportunity, or are not prepared to offer a modified curriculum to special children such as yours. The child is often at the mercy of Normalcy.

YOUR CHILD will probably be delayed in graduating from high school. He will enter the world of occupations at a much later time than the average child of the same age, a loss that can easily be measured in dollars and cents.

YOUR CHILD will be discouraged and runs the chance of becoming an early dropout—or pushout!

The specific area of intelligence measurement where the loss is most obvious is the storage of information, or better, the retrieval of such information. But how can one retrieve if the information has not been stored in the first place? Not even a computer could perform such a feat. By a lowering of intelligence, in terms of IQ scores, we do not mean sheer reasoning power or the ability to conceptualize, for these remain fairly intact in the child. In children with neurological deficiencies or damage, this would be another matter. But if the poor reader with a specific language problem such as dyslexia is not exposed sufficiently to information in his environment, then the measure in this particular area or subtest will gradually go down, unless the same information is given him via perceptual and cognitive routes other than those based on reading material, that is, the printed word.

Can we find ways and means to prevent this loss, or to invent countermeasures? This fatal by-product of a reading problem is quite interesting and often not known to educators and parents, who feel that once a child has been diagnosed and treatment initiated, remediation will have to do the job. A verbatim summary of an article on this subject is quoted here to underline the importance of the matter:

As more children in this country are exposed to education, and for longer periods of time, the number who are encountering difficulty in school increases. For many of these children, the problem is simply that, in order to learn, they must read. For a large number of children with learning problems or IQ's below 100, this requisite artificially deprives them of the comfortable avenues for learning. Modern technology provides equipment to educate many of the children for whom reading is either an uncomfortable or inefficient technique. For such children, a bookless curriculum is proposed which would provide children with an education while reading is relegated to a more realistic role in education, that of a skill area which is only one of the many tools available for learning.[1]

[1] N. E. and M. C. Silberberg, "The Bookless Curriculum: An Educa-

The authors of the article from which the quotation above was taken also state that "in order to learn, a child must read," and go on to say that a child who cannot meet this criterion of reading will not receive knowledge or information but will have to develop the skill of reading *while delaying the rest of the learning experience.* Some educators contend that with the onset of computers and advanced technologies and mechanical devices of all sorts, we might be heading toward a nonreading society, at least in the sense of reading as we know it today. But immediate and present requirements for reading will be with us for some time to come, it appears, and the reading requirements are undeniably with us now while our children are still going to school and have to learn our antiquated ABC's.

Fortunately, compensation in these children can take many forms. While they do not always understand what they read because of faulty perception that distorts the visual image received by the brain, their hearing and comprehension are still intact and function well. They comprehend what they hear, but they do not necessarily comprehend what is presented to them in written form. The reception of further information can reach them via the oral-aural avenues, that is, speaking and hearing. In order for these children to gain further information that is commensurate with their age group and general ability, they must keep up with the world outside and must be fed the vitally needed information—spoon-fed, if necessary—to avoid the terrible shutdown of the gates that lead to the information storage vaults in their brains, a storage of intellectual treasures and common facts which they will have to

180

draw upon in years to come, not just during the testing of their intelligence. Immediate recall of a word or an idea just learned is one thing, but long-range retention and storage is quite another. It is exactly here where these children need help—now.

What can be done about this situation? Here are some practical, down-to-earth suggestions to overcome this cognitive waning, this continual lack of exposure to the information-feeding sources in the written form, such as books, magazines, newspapers, journals, and pamphlets of all sorts. Information in written form obviously implies *reading*. And that is precisely where these children are handicapped for the time being.

Information Feeder Devices and Sources

1. *Oral Reading.* Very similar to the blind, by abhorrent analogy, children with a specific reading disability must be read to every day, every hour, every free minute. They are unable to do the job by themselves. Home assignments in textbooks and workbooks should be read to them *aloud*, and time allowed for them to ask questions for a check on their comprehension of the material. Often it may require special permission from the teacher or principal to have children take home their readers and textbooks. This oral reading may at times be considered a burden on the members of the family; but it is a survival technique and lifesaver of no small consequence and should be carried out to make more and accurate information available to the child.

2. *Tape Recorder.* If it is inconvenient for the members of the family or friends to read to the child at a certain time during the afternoon or at night, the material can be pre-recorded on tape, and the child may listen to the recording

at a time convenient for him. Tape recorders are relatively inexpensive machines, fortunately, and allow for extended playing time, up to several hours if special tape is used. The tape recorder offers a wide variety of uses and possibilities, not only for the reading of home assignments or other sources. Dreaded book reports may first be recorded orally by the child. The writing of essays or brief reports can be an insurmountable chore for these children, but recording a draft orally on tape will help them later to put their thoughts and words in writing. The tape recorder has intrinsic appeal for the child, thus favoring his eagerness to do work that is otherwise painful. Earphones may help him to concentrate more by cutting out extraneous stimuli bombarding him, but such exercises should not be overextended in time.

3. *Phonograph Records.* While we think of records as being reserved for recreational services, there are many educational records available on the commercial market, ranging from the teaching of phonetics and the multiplication tables to foreign languages and events in history. Classical children's literature and rhythm exercises are also available on records. Again here is an excellent mechanical device that can be used to widen the child's access to readily stored information and common knowledge. Public libraries usually have records on free loan as part of their regular services to the community.

4. *Educational Television.* Most localities now are within the viewing area of Educational TV stations. The programs of these stations usually offer a wide and highly interesting variety of lessons and features. It is not necessary that the child watch a particular program at his own grade level, but he should be exposed to many programs within his scope of comprehension and interest. Travelogues, biog-

raphies, plays, or special events features all contain an enormous amount of information vital to the child's academic survival. Strengthening the basic skills by allowing him to watch a program *below* his actual grade level can also be of value. Frequently the ETV stations bring reruns of their weekly fare on Saturdays or during the evening hours.

5. *Films and Filmstrips.* Watching sound films and filmstrips or slides does not necessarily require reading, and they are also an excellent medium for conveying the type of information we have talked about in this connection. Title slides and other written material on film can be read aloud together with the child, time permitting. Not every family has a movie projector, but this is not always necessary. For schools, projectors are of course standard equipment. Frequently libraries in town offer free film shows as part of their service to the public, and their choice of film subjects usually has educational value. Commercial movie houses may also show films which at times contain educational glimpses such as biographical material on certain heroes and famous men. Departments of Recreation may also be of assistance in this connection. Perhaps the reader might even be so persuasive as to have the school put on special film shows, right at the school, for a selected group of children who are in desperate need of this type of additional feeding of information. Perhaps the president of a school's PTA can lend a helping hand, using the organization's influence for a worthwhile cause. Slides are even more accessible than films, and the vast resource of travelers and foreign-born people with interesting slide collections on foreign countries should not be overlooked. Again, libraries have slide collections on loan.

6. *Field Trips.* A child with a specific reading problem should have many opportunities to listen, observe, and look

around, but he should preferably be freed from the painful chains of having to read to gain access to information. Parents and educators must try to make the most out of a trip to the zoo or a visit to a local factory. The child should have ample opportunity to ask questions. If no questions are posed by the child, an attempt should be made to stimulate him into discussing what he has observed. Retention of facts is more effective when verbalized repeatedly. This exposure to incidental learning situations lends itself well to the enrichment of the child's spoken vocabulary and storage of knowledge, information that ardent readers may gather from books and magazines.

7. *Reading Clubs.* Previously it was suggested that reading groups be established to tutor the poor reader in a more formal way. The same suggestion could be useful for forming small groups on the block or from nearby homes where the children could be brought together, as often as possible, for reading sessions. An adult or good reader could read to these groups of poor readers, with subsequent discussions of the material to improve retention and comprehension. The success of the program depends largely on the selection of highly interesting and challenging material. Sometimes it is possible to persuade fathers or male members of the neighborhood to participate in these sessions as readers, lending some prestige and hero worship to the materials being read. It is also feasible to supplement these presentations with slides, if available, or filmstrips and plays.

The list of useful suggestions actually does not end here but should be the creative beginning of what might be called an academic survival program for children with reading disabilities. It does not matter how young or old the child is; in fact, the younger the better, because the preventive aspects of such a program would be of even greater benefit to a youngster with an incipient dyslexic condition.

Some consideration should also be given to proper record keeping during tutorial efforts over a period of time, and to the reinforcement principles in learning. Recently the terms *behavior modification* and *operant conditioning* have crept into educational institutions and classrooms. These techniques are not necessarily new but are now applied to learning situations. The main point in these techniques is the reward system, or reinforcement, which is supposed to tease out of the child's behavioral repertoire already existing desirable behavior, for example, effective learning. Through rewarding this already existing behavior, its frequency can be increased. For example, a child may be able to concentrate on his reading lessons for three to five minutes, but then become restless and bored. It is possible that through effective rewards the child may increase his interest and concentration span. Or the young reader may be rewarded positively with a small token of some kind after a certain amount of reading has been done. The secret here is to isolate a small unit of behavior and consistently reward it on a preplanned basis. Reinforcements can be both positive and negative, and verbal as well as nonverbal. In an educational setting, nonverbal positive rewards seem to prevail in practice, especially with younger children. When a chart is kept for the child as to his daily assignments and accomplishments, stars or check marks could be placed behind the accomplishments of each lesson, session or day, and the child then be rewarded commensurately with his efforts or correct answers. Whole classrooms can be managed in this way.

Finally, what should be of great concern to parents and educators regarding their dyslexic children is the appearance of secondary emotional reactions in response to the primary learning disabilities. The child faces continuous failures while in a regular school setting where reading is at a premium. The poor reader and dyslexic child are constantly given to understand, in one way or another, that they are not meeting the expectations of teacher or parent. The F mark on the report card stands for *Failure*; it is as if the child were ostracized from the very culture in which he lives. Indeed the nonreading child must feel like a blind child in many ways. In due time he will show emotional reactions to this kind of failure, the disrespect from peers and adults, and the continuous agony he must endure. These secondary emotional reactions, as they are called among professionals, may take on severe forms in some instances and be mistaken and misdiagnosed as emotional disturbances of a primary nature, while the dyslexic condition goes unrecognized and untreated.

The subject of secondary emotional reactions to primary and specific learning disabilities will be discussed briefly by first mentioning the developmental-psychological aspects, followed by an overview of some of the therapeutic possibilities available to the child and his family.

Dyslexia and Retention in School

When the failing student with an undetected dyslexic condition keeps falling behind in school, the possibility of retention is often considered by both parents and educators. Repeating a grade might just give the child the added time and opportunity to catch up with his peers. But the decision is not as simple as that. Many things have to be considered, quite aside from the fact that it will cost the school system and the taxpayer a considerable amount of money to hold a child back one year.

When a child is developmentally immature and if this condition has caused the poor academic performance, this author usually does not hesitate to recommend a retention as long as the child is in kindergarten or first grade. Small children do not show any severe reactions to being retained. If the developmental lag is characterized by clumsiness, inarticulate speech, poor visual and auditory perceptions, and so on, repeating a program can be beneficial. However, older children often oppose the retention and do not benefit from this repetition of the same grade, sometimes getting the same teacher and the same books, with no added special help or remedial work. Older children may need the peer group for emotional growth and development much more than the defeat and humiliation of going down a grade and joining children one year younger. At times, especially when more than one year's retention takes place, the child has to join a much younger peer group and shows signs of regression. Promotions with a fortified curriculum and special education placement, such as resource room or tutorial assistance, are more indicated and more helpful. If the child has low intelligence, bordering on slow-learner levels, retention might be more indicated than in bright children with above-average intelligence.

There is no definite rule or yardstick by which one can determine the suitability of a retention. Each child is individually different and deserves the full attention and concern of both parent and educator.

Dyslexia and Delinquency

The relationship of dyslexia to delinquency is often cited as being as high as 80 percent. One must be cautious about making hasty inferences when studying a mere relationship, meaning only that the two variables overlap. The relationship does not allow for conceptual inferences based on statistical manipulations, as every scientist well knows. However, the relationship is nevertheless alarming, to say the least.

In a recent sniper episode in one of the Southern states, the crime of a seventeen-year-old boy was vividly described. A terse paragraph at the end of the article mentioned, almost parenthically, the fact that the youth "had received special education for dyslexia, or reading difficulties, which had kept him from attending regular classes for a year."

Delinquency may perhaps be the result of a poor self-image and continuous failure. But why are not all dyslexic children criminally inclined? Apparently we don't have the full answer yet. In a research study reported in the *Journal of Counseling Psychology* (Vol. 6, 1952), E. Ellis Graham examined ninety-six "unsuccessful readers" and compared their scores on an intelligence test with those obtained by children having "psychopathic profiles." The ages of these children ranged from eight to sixteen years. In discussing his results, Graham mentions that their scattergrams (profiles based on several subtests of intelligence) correspond closely with those described by others doing research with the adolescent psychopath. He adds that if the unsuccessful reader is unconsciously *resisting* the emotional climate of the school or home, this should be expected. However, if the resistance is passive, there may be no other noticeable trouble. If it is active, it might well manifest itself in truancy and other violations of authority or the law. This explanation, even though perhaps in a speculative vein, is about the best we can offer, since the dyslexic child still remains a puzzle in this respect. It points up one important inference:

If the dyslexic child remains untreated, we can expect more trouble. If intervention is instigated and remedial help offered, there is hope.

Essential Ingredients of a Survival Program

Remedial procedures have been outlined in this book in previous chapters and need no repetition here. Suffice it to say that the best intervention we can procure is that of professionally trained persons. If that is unavailable, *survival techniques* are a must to assuage the dyslexic's anxieties and apprehensions. Here are some *musts*:

1. *15-Minute Tutorial Sessions.* The parent or a suitable surrogate must sit with the child every night for 15 minutes and teach him on a one-to-one basis in an emotionally unexplosive climate. If no other techniques are available, the parent and child can sit side by side and read out loud together—in chorus, as it were. This is a proved method (neurological impress method) that has built-in correctional features. It teaches pronunciation and rhythm, and provides feedback. The secret here is to conduct these sessions consistently and systematically every day, rain or shine, holiday or not. It does not matter if the sessions are not always carried out at a specific time of the day or night, as long as they are carried out every day. A calendar on the wall can serve as a reminder, and the child may be asked to make a check mark on it every day, after the session is completed. This will also serve as a reinforcer. After a series of sessions— say five or ten—the child is offered a small reward for good attendance.

2. *Perceptual Problems.* If the child has perceptual problems manifested in his inability to copy simple designs, or left-right confusion revealed in reversal errors in reading (*d*

for *b*, or *was* for *saw*), simple copying exercises are essential and have been described elsewhere in this book. Simple graph paper is suitable for these exercises because a blank sheet of paper causes confusion in orientation on the page. These children need *structure*, and graph paper provides for such structural orientation on the page. If the child copies designs incorrectly, corrections are made by *telling* and *showing* him how to do it, without the parent's resorting to deprecating remarks. The situation must be pleasant for both child and parent. Reinforcement can be provided by asking the child to trace his good copy designs with a felt-tip pen.

3. *Tactile-Kinesthetic Approach.* Our 15-minute survival sessions must include the application of the tactile-kinesthetic technique, in which the child traces letters and words on a rough surface (sand tray, tabletop, sandpaper, rug, or in Southern states, grits!). This technique is best applied when spelling is taught. Most children have spelling words as their daily or weekly assignments. Before requiring the child to write down the words, he should be asked to write them on a rough surface *three times*, and then make his first attempt to write them on a sheet of paper. The words are also written on a 3-by-five-inch index card, and at the beginning of each new session the child goes over those words, placed in front of him in a stack. The cards that are correctly read or spelled go in one pile, and the cards with which the child still experiences difficulty go in another. Obviously, the incorrectly read or spelled cards need further reinforcement by writing the words again on a tabletop.

4. *Phonetic/Auditory Exercises.* If a child has difficulty with phonetics in school, remediation is needed for survival. After all, the English language is approximately 70 percent

phonetic, and if we fail to get any phonetic clues in our reading, efficiency is greatly reduced and the child depends exclusively on visual clues. Auditory difficulties reveal themselves in not hearing the difference between sounds, like *pet* and *pit*, provided they are properly pronounced by the model speaker. Children may also have difficulty with translating a sound they hear into the symbol the sound stands for, like the "huh" sound and the "H" letter that symbolically represents the sound. Of course, sometimes we have complications, as when the "fuh" sound is represented by either "F" or "PH."

The reader may wish to look up the section in this book that deals with auditory discrimination, in which a simple "beeper" or telegraph key is employed for the auditory training.* It is important that a child who has relative phonetic insensitivity be trained first in more fundamental skills, such as auditory discrimination training, without resorting to letters and words. This can be done by using dots and dashes (for example, . . – . .) as the basic symbolism, rather than the more complicated linguistic symbols (alphabet).

5. *Supportive Counseling.* The tutorial, one-to-one relationship is highly inducive to a calm atmosphere in which concerns can be talked over with an empathic listener. Any tutorial situation has this built-in counseling technique. In cases where secondary emotional reactions have taken the upper hand, more intensive counseling is needed to hold adjustment at as normal a level as possible. The school counselor and a professional psychologist may have to be

---

* For gamelike exercises in phonetic training, see R. F. Wagner, *Teaching Phonics with Success* (Johnstown, Pa.: Mafex Associates, 1960).

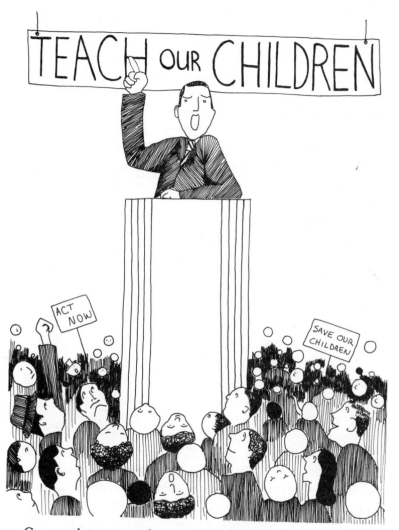

Concerned parents and assertive citizens can do much for our handicapped children by seeking the cooperation of school administrators. (Illustration by Whitney Hardy)

employed here, or the services of community resources, especially mental health clinics and guidance centers, may have to be explored in search of suitable counselors.

Survival techniques are exactly what the term implies: they can serve only as an interim procedure until—one hopes—more adequate and professional services can be located. Often the exercises can at least prevent the dyslexic condition from becoming worse.

The dilemma of the dyslexic child is not over, but great strides are being made toward more effective and frequent help for them. In this connection, *parent power* should not be overlooked. Many a school system has reviewed its services to the learning-disabled child and, more often than not, come up with new programs and extended services after concerned and determined parents as well as interested, assertive citizens have approached the school administrators. We now have good laws to protect the rights of our handicapped children, but *people* must guard the laws and make them a reality.

APPENDIX A · RECOMMENDED READING

After reading this book, the reader may wish to deepen or widen his knowledge of the subject of learning disabilities or obtain further information by seeking the opinion of other authors or facts from other sources. The following list of books and publications is very selective and was compiled in an attempt to pick out more informative and semitechnical sources of information. While the author has tried to retain a sense of objectivity, certain publications were not included, especially when the contents are tendentious, one-sided, or highly controversial.

Books

Barsch, R. H. A Movigenic Curriculum. Madison, Wis.: Bureau for Handicapped Children, 1965. Deals primarily with sensorimotor exercises for younger children in need of coordination training.

Critchley, M. The Dyslexic Child. Springfield, Ill.: Charles C. Thomas, 1970.

Cruickshank, W. M., et al. A Teaching Method for Brain-Injured and Hyperactive Children. Syracuse, N.Y.: Syracuse University Press, 1961.

DeHirsch, Katrina, et al. Predicting Reading Failure. New York: Harper & Row, 1966.

Frostig, M., and Horne, D. The Frostig Program for the Development of Visual Perception. Chicago: Follett, 1964.

Gillingham, A., and Stillman, B. Remedial Training for Children with Specific Disabilities in Reading, Spelling, and Penmanship. Cambridge, Mass.: Educators Publishing Co., 1960.

Hammill, D. D., and Bartel, N. R. Educational Perspectives in Learning Disabilities. New York: Wiley, 1974.

Heckelman, R. G. "Using the Neurological Impress Remedial Reading Techniques," Academic Therapy, Summer 1966, pp. 235–239.

Huey, Edmund B. The Psychology and Pedagogy of Reading. Cambridge, Mass.: M.I.T. Press, 1968.

Johnson, D. J., and Myklebust, H. P. Learning Disabilities. New York: Grune and Stratton, 1967.

Kirk, S. Diagnosis and Remediation of Learning Disabilities. Urbana: University of Illinois Press, 1966.

Kirk, S., and Kirk, W. Psycholinguistic Learning Disabilities: Diagnosis and Remediation. Urbana: University of Illinois Press, 1971.

Lerner, J. W. *Children with Learning Disabilities: Theories, Diagnosis, and Teaching Strategies.* Boston: Houghton Mifflin, 1971.

Money, John (ed.) *The Disabled Reader.* Baltimore, Md.: The Johns Hopkins University Press, 1966.

Orton, S. *Reading, Writing, and Speech Problems in Children.* New York: Norton, 1937. Available from Educators Publishing Co., Cambridge, Mass.

Rawson, Margaret B. *Developmental Language Disability, Adult Accomplishments of Dyslexic Boys.* Baltimore, Md.: The Johns Hopkins University Press, 1968.

Strauss, A., and Lehtinen, L. *Psychopathology and Education of the Brain-Injured Child.* New York: Grune and Stratton, 1947.

Tarnopol, L. (ed.) *Learning Disabilities: Introduction to Educational and Medical Management.* Springfield, Ill.: Charles C. Thomas, 1969.

Wagner, R. F. *Helping the Wordblind: Effective Intervention Techniques for Overcoming Reading Problems in Older Students.* West Nyack, N.Y.: Center for Applied Research in Education, 1976.

———. *Teaching Phonics with Success.* Johnstown, Pa.: Mayfex Associates, 1960, 1969.

Professional Journals

Relevant articles on the subject of learning disabilities can be found in many journals and magazines of a professional nature, as well as in the more popular women's magazines and similar publications. The journals named below specialize in the subject of learning disabilities.

Academic Therapy Quarterly. The journal covers a wide range of subjects related to learning disabilities and also contains a special section for parents. Besides the journal, the company also publishes materials, tests, and books on the same subject, some of them reprints from the journal. Catalog upon request by writing to Academic Therapy Publications, 28 Commercial Blvd., Novato, Calif. 94947. Four issues yearly. Special summer editions list schools available throughout the United States, including camps for dyslexics.

Bulletin of the Orton Society. An interdisciplinary journal of specific language disability (dyslexia), published annually by the Orton Society, National Headquarters, Suite 115, 8415 Bellona Lane, Towson, Md. 21204. Has international contributors.

Journal of Learning Disabilities. A journal with multidisciplinary contributors to the field of learning disabilities. International in character, it includes a practical section for teachers and parents, information on books and relevant literature in the field, and information on current legal matters on the national scene. Order from *Journal of Learning Disabilities,* 101 East Ontario St., Chicago, Ill. 60611. Monthly issues, by subscription only.

Learning Disabilities Guide. Not labeled as a journal, this loose-leaf-type guide is published nine times per year by subscription. Separate editions for elementary and secondary levels. Primarily for teachers. Croft NEI Publications, 24 Rope Ferry Road, Waterford, Conn. 06386.

Perceptions. A newsletter for parents of children with learning disabilities, this bulletin-type publication is published eight times a year, monthly, except for July, August, December, and January. Contains information especially for parents, such as new laws, meetings, remedial tips, etc. Write to: Perceptions, Inc., P.O. Box 142, Millburn, N.J. 07041.

Readings in Learning Disabilities. The Special Learning Corporation produces soft-cover volumes on an annual or biannual basis containing a collection of the more important professional articles on the subject of learning disabilities. The company also publishes the same type of format on other handicaps; for example, dyslexia. Special Learning Corporation, 42 Boston Post Road, Guilford, Conn. 06437.

Professional Associations

There are several organizations on the national and state level that concern themselves with children's learning disabilities and related topics. Since these children go under various labels—neurologically handicapped, minimal brain dysfunction, brain-damaged, dyslexic, legasthenic, and so on—no one organization has assumed sole responsibility for them. Among the better-known associations in the field of learning disabilities are the following:

Association for Children with Learning Disabilities. (ACLD). The association is particularly interested in furthering the cause of children with specific learning disabilities. The national office is located in Pittsburgh, Pa., and has affiliated state and local chapters in almost all states as well as some affiliations abroad. For a complete list of state offices and their current presidents (including addresses), the reader may write to the association headquarters: Association for Children with Learning Disabilities, 4156 Library Road, Pittsburgh, Pa. 15234. Telephone: 412-341-1515. The association also has books for sale (request a complete book list) and holds annual conferences and conventions at the national, state, and local levels.

California Association for Neurologically Handicapped Children. The association was founded in California but reaches much farther into geographical sections of the country. Address: California Association for Neurologically Handicapped Children (CANHC), P.O. Box 4088, Los Angeles, Calif. 90051. The organization issues helpful lists on publications pertaining to learning disabilities and related topics (write to Literature Distribution Center, P.O. Box 1526, Vista, Calif. 92083) as well as a directory of films relative to learning disabilities (address the CANHC, 645 Odin Drive, Pleasant Hill, Calif. 94523).

Canadian Association for Children with Learning Disabilities. The association has a chapter in nearly every province in Canada and helps parents to find professional help, recommends books and pamphlets on learning disabilities, and puts inquiring people in touch with other parents who have coped with similar problems. Address: Canadian Association for Children with Learning Disabilities, 88 Eglinton Avenue East, Toronto 315, Ontario, Canada.

Closer Look. This is a government-sponsored organization serving parents and professionals seeking information about organizations, legal rights, and resources for parents regarding learning disabilities and related topics and conditions. Address: Closer Look, Box 1492, Washington, D.C. 20013.

Council for Exceptional Children (CEC). CEC is the professional organization for all special educators. It also serves as a clearinghouse for the handicapped as well as gifted and offers many information services. For example, topical bibliographies of professional resources, journal articles, curriculum guides, and program descriptions are available from this source. For further information, write: Council for Exceptional Children, 1920 Association Drive, Reston, Va. 22091.

National Information Center on Special Education Materials (NICSEM). Located at the University of Southern California, University Park, Los Angeles, Calif. 90007. NICSEM is a project funded by the Bureau of Education for the Handicapped to provide information about instructional materials and resources useful in the education of handicapped individuals.

The Orton Society, Inc. This is a nonprofit scientific and educational organization for the study and treatment of children with specific language disability (dyslexia). Founded in honor of Dr. Samuel T. Orton, the Orton Society does not espouse or prescribe any "official" system or systems of remedial education. The membership fee includes a subscription to the *Bulletin of the Orton Society,* published annually. The society also holds annual conventions throughout the United States. Address: The Orton Society, National Headquarters, Suite 115, 8415 Bellona Lane, Towson, Md. 21204. The society has several branches distributed throughout the United States. All branches hold at least one public meeting or workshop per year.

APPENDIX B · GLOSSARY OF TERMS

AGNOSIA: The inability to identify objects through the senses; for example, finger agnosia.

ALPHA RHYTHM: One of the several rhythms found in the brain as recorded and amplified by the EEG (electro-encephalograph, or brain-wave test). It consists of rhythmic activity between 8 and 12 hertz (cycles per second). There are also beta, theta, and delta rhythms.

AUDITORY CLOSURE: The ability to find the "missing" sound in a sequence of sounds; for example, micro—one (microphone).

AUDITORY DISCRIMINATION: The ability to differentiate between and among different sounds, in isolation or sequence; for example, the difference between *pit* and *pet*.

AUDITORY SEQUENTIAL MEMORY: The ability to reproduce in correct sequence what was perceived through the ears (hearing); for example, a series of digits (6, 4, 8, 9).

APHASIA: The loss or the impairment of the ability to express oneself through speech or writing (receptive or expressive loss, or mixed type). There is a distinction between sensory aphasia (input) and expressive aphasia (output).

BODY IMAGE: The awareness of one's body as it relates to movement, space, or surrounding objects. Children with neurological damage frequently have difficulty in this area, which also shows up in their drawings of the human figure.

CATASTROPHIC REACTION: An extreme reaction to changes in relative routine, unexpected events, overstimulation, or frustration. Children may throw objects, destroy their own work, or burst into tantrums or tears.

CEREBRAL: Relating to the brain.

COGNITIVE FUNCTIONS: The intellectual or thinking functions of the brain.

DEXTRALITY: Right-sidedness, especially with reference to right-handedness.

DISTRACTIBILITY: A shifting of attention from the task at hand to distracting stimuli in the environment, such as light, sound, or moving objects. The child gives too much attention to these irrelevant stimuli and therefore cannot concentrate.

DYSCALCULIA: A partial inability to do arithmetic; a learning disability relating to numerical concepts and mathematical reasoning.

DYSEIDEDIC DYSLEXIA: In dyseidedic dyslexia, the child has difficulty in perceiving words as wholes and reads phonetically. Misspellings are phonetic; for example, *lisn* for *listen*.

DYSGRAPHIA: The inability to write legibly, implying difficulty with loops, letter sequence, or slanting. Hans Christian Andersen was a prime example of a dysgraphic.

DYSLEXIA: A partial inability to read in a person of normal and above-normal intelligence including children. A specific learning disability focusing on reading. The term was coined by Dr. Rudolf Berlin, an ophthalmologist of Stuttgart, Germany.

DYSPHONETIC DYSLEXIA: Dysphonetic dyslexia is characterized by deficits in sound integration because of lack of phonetic sensitivity. Mistakes are often substitutions, such as *chicken* for *duck*.

EEG: The electroencephalogram, or brain-wave test, which records and amplifies the rhythms of the brain.

ETIOLOGY: The cause of a disability or disease.

GERSTMANN'S SYNDROME: A complex disorder of brain functions accompanied by lesions giving rise to right-left disorientation, finger agnosia, dysgraphia, and dyscalculia.

GESTALT: Configuration, form, or totality (from the German).

HYPERACTIVITY: Abnormal motor activity; behavior characterized by continual motion; for example, fidgeting in a chair, drumming the fingers, tapping the feet.

HYPERKINESIS: The medical term for hyperactivity.

HYPOACTIVITY: Abnormal motor activity, at the opposite extreme from hyperactivity; that is, inactivity.

INCOORDINATION: A behavior characterized by physical awkwardness and unusual clumsiness, sometimes affecting eye-hand coordination.

LABILE: Unstable, as referring to emotional adjustment; for example, vacillating behavior, the inability to make decisions.

LATERALITY: Sidedness, especially with regard to hands, eyes, and feet as the preferred or dominant side; for example, right-handedness.

LESION: A structural or functional alteration in the brain, due to an injury.

LOOK-SAY METHOD: Learning to read only by looking and saying; the word-recognition method.

MINIMAL BRAIN DYSFUNCTION: Abbreviated MBD or MCD (minimal cerebral dysfunction); a medical term referring to children with mild to severe learning or behavior problems, with at least normal intellectual functioning, assuming deviations in brain functions due to illness or injury. The etiology is often unknown.

MIXED CEREBRAL
DOMINANCE:
Also referred to as *crossed
dominance pattern*; the assumption that one-half of the brain (one cerebral hemisphere) is controlling an act of behavior, thus introducing confusion. Example: Left handed, right-eyed, left-footed. Behavioral act is *not* unilaterally controlled.

NEUROPSYCHOLOGY:
A specialized branch of psychology, dealing with the neurological aspects of psychological behavior.

OPERANT BEHAVIOR:
A behavior whose rate or form is affected by its consequences; also associated with behavior-modification techniques (conditioning) to control the behavior of children. *Token economy* is the term used when groups are involved, receiving tokens as rewards for good behavior.

OPHTHALMOLOGIST:
A physician specializing in the diseases of the eye.

OTOLOGIST:
A physician specializing in the diseases of the ear; often an ENT (ear-nose-throat) specialist.

PEDAGOGY:
Principles and methods of teaching children.

PERSEVERATION:
The tendency to continue an activity, often related to brain dysfunction or mental subnor-

mality; for example, continuing to make dots in a line on paper to the edge, without the ability to stop. Repetitive behavior.

PHONETIC: Referring to speech sounds; or the sounding out of written symbols.

REVERSAL: The tendency to reverse letters, numbers, and words in reading; for example, reading *was* for *saw*, or saying *14* for *41*. Sometimes called *mirror reading*.

ROTE MEMORY: Reproduction of learned material in which the factor of meaning is disregarded.

SCHOOL PHOBIA: The irrational fear in children of going to school, in the absence of real threats.

TACTILE APPROACH: The tracing of words by children with dyslexia or other difficulties in learning; usually done with the finger in sand or on a rough surface. Also known as the *tactile-kinesthetic approach*.

VISUAL CLOSURE: The ability to identify an object from an incomplete presentation; finding the "missing part" to make the whole.

VISUAL DISCRIMINATION: The ability to distinguish between or among different letters or words; for example, between *b* and *d*.

VISUAL PERCEPTION: The visual structuring of the field as a prerequisite to comprehension.

WAIS: The Wechsler Adult Intelligence Scale, an intelligence test.

WISC: The Wechsler Intelligence Scale for Children; also the WISC-R, the revised version of the WISC.